Our Aging Bodies

Our Aging Bodies

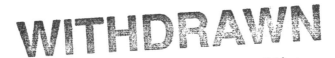

GARY F. MERRILL

RUTGERS UNIVERSITY PRESS

NEW BRUNSWICK, NEW JERSEY, AND LONDON

LIBRARY OF CONGRESS CATALOGING-IN-PUBLICATION DATA

Merrill, Gary F., author.
    Our aging bodies / Gary F. Merrill.
        p. ; cm.
    Includes index.
    ISBN 978–0–8135–7156–0 (hardcover: alk. paper) — ISBN 978–0–8135–7155–3
(pbk. : alk. paper) — ISBN 978–0–8135–7157–7 (e-book)
    I. Title.
    [DNLM: 1. Aging—physiology. WT 104]
    QP86
    612.6′7—dc23   2014016470

A British Cataloging-in-Publication record for this book is available
from the British Library.

Visit our website: http://rutgerspress.rutgers.edu

Manufactured in the United States of America

CONTENTS

ACKNOWLEDGMENTS

I acknowledge the kindness and professionalism of everyone at Rutgers University Press, especially Dana Dreibelbus, executive editor for health and medicine. I also acknowledge my wife, Marlene, and all those who like her are aging with grace and silence.

Our Aging Bodies

1

How We Age

Dorland's Illustrated Medical Dictionary defines aging as "the gradual changes in the structure of an organism that occur with the passage of time, that do not result from disease or other gross accidents and that eventually lead to the increased probability of death as the individual grows older." Following this definition, *Dorland's* refers the reader to the word "senescence." I would modify *Dorland's* definition slightly by adding the words "and function" after the word "structure."

Currently, there are nearly 500 million people sixty years and older in the world, and by 2030 this population will double to one billion. Increasingly, the preponderance of older people will reside in developing countries where fertility rates have declined markedly, accompanied by reduced mortality. For instance, there will be 370 million older adults living in China and India alone by 2030. However, not only is the overall population aging, but the older population is getting older as well. In the United States, for example, the oldest old (people eighty-five years and older) is the most rapidly growing segment of the population. This group will quadruple to 21 million people by 2050, at which time one out of every four older adults is projected to be eighty-five years or older.

Since the second half of the twentieth century, many countries have witnessed the increased graying of their populations. Japan currently has the largest proportion of people aged sixty-five years and older, at 23 percent. That is projected to rise to 40 percent by the year 2050. In the United States, 12 percent of the population currently consists of older adults, a

proportion that is projected to rise to 20 percent by the year 2050. Similarly, older adults comprise 21 percent of the current population of the
European Union, with Sweden and Italy having the largest numbers of old
people. The elderly proportion of the European population is projected to
equal that of Japan by 2050 due to phenomenal steady declines in the birth
rates for Japan and for the European Union. Demographic shifts toward the
increasing numbers of elderly people are not occurring exclusively in
industrialized countries; they are a global phenomenon. Older adults are
projected to constitute up to 25 and 15 percent, respectively, of the aggregate population of developed and least developed countries by 2050.
Considering the myriad age-related physiological alterations and the
projected steady rise in the cost of geriatric medical care in every country,
the aging of the world population is a pandemic that presents biomedical,
socioeconomic, and geopolitical challenges.

This is a book about aging and its influences on the body's major
organ systems. It is not a book about aging-related diseases, which is a different topic for another writer. Chapter 1 is an introductory chapter. Here
I write about role models in aging, documented cases from the late twentieth and early twenty-first centuries of the oldest and healthiest among us.
Perhaps the countries, provinces, regions, and states they live in have contributed to their longevity, and we will learn how this happened at some
future date. In this chapter I also write of some of the unavoidable facts of
aging, such as coming of age politically and socially, aging prematurely,
and anxiety and premature aging. I include thoughts on diet, physical
activity, and the role of humor in aging. Finally, this chapter concludes
with a discussion of current theories about how and why we get old and
about the proposed mechanisms that cause aging. All of this should help
readers understand their own longevity and some of the trials and challenges that await them.

My family, friends, and I are aging. I'm reminded of this when I have
lunch each semester with retired colleagues, spend time at triannual family reunions, or unexpectedly bump into former neighbors around town.
Another reminder is our family room. It is a photo gallery of five generations of family members. On separate walls my wife, an excellent photog-
rapher and repository of family history, has displayed pictures of our
grandchildren, children, parents, and grandparents. She and I are the third

of the five generations pictured there. It is a rare visitor who does not take time to examine these photos and ask questions. On one occasion when my teaching assistants were invited to dinner in our home, a few of the young women were looking at the photos. Pointing to a picture of my maternal grandfather, they asked my wife if that was my father. This was the first time I recall anyone suggesting that resemblance. I had never considered myself to look like that grandfather. To the right of his photograph, and one row below, is a picture of my parents. I and most other visitors (including my siblings) think I look like my father, but these three young women thought my resemblance to my father was weaker than that to my maternal grandfather. Beauty (or at least resemblance) truly is in the eyes of the beholder.

I look at those pictures each time I am relaxing in our family room. All the photographs of our parents and grandparents were taken at or near the times of their weddings. Without exception, the women ranged in age from about seventeen to twenty-five. The men were three to ten years older than their wives. I believe our parents and grandparents look much older in those photos than they actually were. For example, if I was a stranger and didn't know the circumstances, I would guess our grandmothers to be in their mid-thirties to late forties at the time the photos were taken. When I look at our mothers, who were seventeen and eighteen at marriage, I believe their hairstyles and other features make them look to be in their mid-to-late twenties. In the photograph of us my wife, who married me at about the same age our mothers were married, looks like the beautiful teenager she was when we met. To me she does not look ten to twenty years older, like our mothers and grandmothers.

My point is that the two generations that preceded ours look to me more aged than they actually were. Most of our grandparents were born between the mid-1890s and about 1905. At that time life expectancies in the United States and Western Europe (where those grandparents were born) for men and women were about fifty years. I am certain that daily living for them was more difficult than it has been for us at corresponding ages. My chopping wood and keeping it stacked neatly in the front porch of my maternal grandparents' small wood-framed house during winter months are among my fondest childhood memories. Waking on cold winter mornings in the mountains of western Wyoming to the smell of that wood burning in a potbellied stove evokes similarly fond memories. My grandfather rose by 5:00 A.M. to whittle kindling and start those fires. My grandmother used that wood and a similar stove and oven for much of her cooking, baking, and warming water to do the dishes. Their lives were spent mostly doing manual labor such as logging, farming, gardening, and sewing and knitting clothes. Some of our grandparents or parents did not go beyond elementary school, and my mother-in-law was the only one in the group to graduate from high school. There was no talk of college or expectation that children would obtain diplomas from universities. My mother's youngest brother attended college for a few semesters but did not graduate. Such was life and aging for my most recent ancestors.

Role Models in Aging

The number of people aged 100 and over has doubled in the United States since 1990 and is sixteen times the number in 1950. Many of these individuals are remarkably fit. When the list of Wisconsin's platoon of centenarians was made public a few years ago, there were fifty-two entries—forty-seven women and five men (that is, women made up 90.4 percent of the group, while men were only 9.6 percent). The earliest date of birth I could find for that group was 1897. The New England Centenarian Study at Boston University Medical Center has found that 25 percent of 169 subjects 100 years of age and older were completely free of significant cognitive disorders and even surpassed the investigators on some mental tests. Fifteen percent lived independently at home, and some were still gainfully employed. Sadly (or happily, depending on your perspective), medical expenses for these subjects were significantly lower than for Americans in their sixties and seventies, and—unlike so many of the rest of us—most centenarians are uncommonly healthy until the very end of their lives. The United Kingdom recently reported that there were nearly 13,000 people aged 100 and over living there (table 1–1).

Stories from the lives of our oldest neighbors are worth telling. Here are a couple of examples. "So what," said Sarah Knauss nearly fifteen years ago, when told that she was the world's oldest living person. Knauss relinquished that title on December 31, 1999, when she died at the age of 119. She had lived through seven US wars, the sinking of the *Titanic*, and

TABLE 1-1

Estimated UK Population Aged 100 Years and Over, 1970–2010

Region	1970	1980	1990	2000	2010
England and Wales	1,080	2,280	4,030	6,230	11,610
Scotland	80	150	260	480	820
Northern Ireland	30	70	100	140	210
UK (total)	1,190	2,500	4,390	6,850	12,640

Source: UK Office for National Statistics.

Charles Lindbergh's solo flight across the Atlantic. She was older than the Brooklyn Bridge and the Statue of Liberty and was already eighty-eight when Neil Armstrong walked on the moon in July 1969. Knauss died in the Phoebe-Devitt Homes Foundation nursing home in Allentown, Pennsylvania, where she had lived for nine years. Born September 24, 1880, in the small coal-mining town of Hollywood, Pennsylvania, she married Abraham Lincoln Knauss in 1901. He became a well-known Republican leader in Lehigh County, Pennsylvania. Sarah was a homemaker and insurance office manager. When her daughter, Kathryn Sullivan, was ninety-six, she explained Knauss's three-digit age by saying: "She's a very tranquil person and nothing fazes her. That's why she's living this long." In 1995, when asked if she enjoyed her long life, Knauss said matter-of-factly: "I enjoy it because I have my health and I can do things." Her passions were said to be watching golf on television, doing needlepoint, and nibbling on milk chocolate turtles, cashews, and potato chips. "Sarah was an elegant lady and worthy of all the honor and adulation she has received," said Joseph Hess, an administrator of the facility where Knauss died quietly in her room. Officials said she had not been ill. She inherited the "oldest" crown, validated by the *Guinness Book of World Records*, with the death of Marie-Louise Febronie Meilleur of Corbeil, Canada, on April 16, 1998. Meilleur had been Knauss's senior by twenty-six days. Neither Knauss nor Meilleur set a longevity record. According to *Guinness*, France's Jeanne Calment, Meilleur's immediate predecessor in the title role, was 122 when she died August 4, 1997.

When Walter Breuning was born he could expect to live about forty years, and he did. Then he lived another forty, and at his death had nearly tripled his life expectancy. Many people had wanted an interview with Breuning, but no one wanted to travel all the way to Great Falls, Montana, to talk to him, a condition set by Breuning. Steve Hartman of *CBS News* was the exception. Hartman reasoned that at age 112, the oldest man in America deserved to have people come to him. The fact that he was alive, cognizant, and mobile at the time is what made an interview with Breuning so valuable (he died in April 2012). Frequently, by the time people reach their mid-eighties, their cognition is so impaired they cannot be interviewed. Not so with Breuning, who could answer your questions and still remembered his grandfather's comments about serving in the Civil War. At his death, Breuning was the only American male still living who was born during the Cleveland administration. He could tell you what he was doing when President William McKinley was shot, and where he attended school when Theodore Roosevelt was president. In the Taft administration, Breuning got a job with the railroad that paid three times less per week than the current minimum wage per hour. He volunteered to serve in World War I but was not called up to fight, and by the time World War II rolled around he was too old to serve. Breuning was married for thirty-five years, but his wife, Agnes, died without having children. Walter never remarried. He said: "Second marriages never work. Even first marriages don't work today." At the time of his interview, Breuning was residing in an assisted living center (although he needed little or no assistance) and went out on errands once each week if the weather was cooperative. "I go to the store and bank," he explained. Other than a modest hearing impairment, Breuning was in near-perfect health. He was taking no medications, was careful about what he ate, and credited his longevity to diet.

Without too much effort one can find data such as those maintained by the Los Angeles Gerontology Research Group for the known super-centenarians of the world. This organization defines a supercentenarian as a validated centenarian who has attained the age of 110 years or more. As of May 9, 2012, there were seventy-one documented supercentenarians—sixty-six women and five men (that is, 93 percent and 7 percent, respectively). They lived in eleven industrialized nations. More than half (thirty-seven) lived in Japan or the United States. Wikipedia reports similar data. As of August 21, 2013, its list included sixty supercentenarians, all but two of whom were women.

The Fundamentals of Aging

Life expectancy in developed nations increased in the twentieth century, and biomedical scientists and governments paid little attention to the change. For example, in the United States life expectancy for males in 1900 was about forty-eight years. That number had increased to about seventy-five years at the beginning of the twenty-first century and is slowly increasing. Similarly, women born in the United States in 1900 had a life expectancy of about fifty-one years, which had increased to about eighty years at the beginning of the twenty-first century. The US National Institutes of Health did not establish the National Institute on Aging until 1974. In 1900 the fraction of the US population sixty-five years or older was only 4 percent. In 2000 it was above 13 percent. Despite the role of antibiotics and other medical advances of the twentieth century, improvements in medicine and health care are not the explanations for this change in demographics of age in the United States during that period. The major explanation is the marked decline in the birth rate, which has accelerated since the 1960s. The reluctance of baby boomers and subsequent generations to have children has caused the elderly to become an increasingly larger fraction of the population. I will forever be grateful that my ancestor Nathaniel Merrill chose to get married and have a family.

Merrill arrived in the American colonies from Ipswich, England, in 1636. He helped settle Ipswich, Massachusetts, then moved to the Hartford, Connecticut, area. His descendants subsequently settled in New York, Michigan, Illinois, Utah, Idaho, and Wyoming, among other locations. I was born in Wyoming. My oldest and youngest sons were born in Utah (1968) and New Jersey (1989), respectively. Even though they have the same parents and were raised in the same family, these two sons arguably belong to different generations. Wikipedia classifies recent American generations differently than I do here. Its classification also differs from that of William Strauss and Neil Howe, experts on the subject. According to Strauss and Howe, I was born at the leading edge of the baby boomer generation (whose first births were in January 1946 and last in December

1963). My parents are members of the so-called silent generation—a name they were given in part because of their political inactivity. According to Strauss and Howe the silent generation (or the greatest generation, according to Tom Brokaw) never produced a US president, but its members volunteered by the millions for military and related service during World War II. After the war ended in 1945, they returned home to a grateful nation. Quietly and without fanfare they got married; had families; and pursued the American dream of home ownership, employment, and security. Their patriotism and work ethic were shaped by their parents' generation, the GI generation. It was so named because some of its members fought in the trenches of World War I, then returned as officers and leaders during World War II. My generation, at 76 million the largest ever, stands in marked contrast to either of its immediate predecessors. We have already produced three US presidents (Bill Clinton, first elected in 1992; George W. Bush, 2000; and Barack Obama, 2008) and will probably produce several more.

Like definitions of generations, measurements of age are simple for the average person to understand but contentious and difficult for the investigators who spend their lives studying the topics. For example, we see a stranger and think to ourselves, "She looks about forty-five." We see childlike behavior in adults and say, "He's acting like a two-year-old." Everyone knows what these expressions mean and can use them correctly. I think my wife looks many years younger than me. Most who have seen us would probably agree, even though we were born only eighteen months apart. Biogerontologists (people who study aging) would say the processes of aging are occurring slowly in my wife and are on schedule or accelerated for me. Biogerontologists also distinguish physiological age from chronological age. Someone can look forty but actually be sixty. When I am physically active, eating a healthy diet, and getting sufficient sleep—that is, when I am at the top of my game—my physiological age seems much younger than my chronological age.

Aging Prematurely

Premature aging syndrome (also called Hutchinson-Gilford Syndrome, progeria of childhood, progeria, and Hutchinson-Gilford Progeria Syndrome) is an extremely rare condition in which some aspects of aging are greatly accelerated, and few children with the syndrome live past their late teens (the character J. F. Sebastian in the 1982 movie *Blade Runner* suffers from progeria). Progeria was first described in 1886 by Jonathan Hutchinson. It was also described, independently, by Hastings Gilford in 1897. About one in eight million babies are born with the disease, although one study from the Netherlands has shown an incidence of one in four million births. It is a genetic condition, but it occurs sporadically and is not inherited. Scientists are particularly interested in progeria because it reveals clues about the normal process of aging. The earliest symptoms include failure to thrive. Children with progeria have a normal appearance in early infancy, but by eight to twenty-four months of age they experience profound delays in growth that lead to diminutive stature and low body weight. They usually have distinctive facial features: a small face-to-head ratio, an underdeveloped jaw (a condition called micrognathia), crowding and unusual form of the teeth, disproportionately large and prominent eyes, a small nose, and a subtle blue hue around the mouth that is indicative of reduced blood flow. In addition, by the second year of life they lose their eyebrows, and eyelashes are lost. This condition—the absence of body hair where it normally grows—is called alopecia. Later small, downy white or blond hairs might grow on the scalp. Other phenotypic (body structure and external appearance) and genotypic (resulting from the composition of genes) characteristics include generalized atherosclerosis; cardiovascular disease and stroke; hip dislocations and stiffness of the joints, along with other defects of the skeletal structure; unusually prominent veins of the scalp; loss of subcutaneous tissue (the layer of fat and other soft tissue beneath the skin and underlying muscle); and defects of the nails.

Children with premature aging syndrome develop early and widespread thickening and loss of elasticity of artery walls (arteriosclerosis). Thickening of the vessel wall, or an increase in the ratio of wall thickness to the vessel's diameter, leads to increased vascular resistance and decreased blood flow, which can worsen until it causes death. During life these changes cause tissue ischemia (insufficient blood flow), reduced delivery of oxygen, and general unavailability of blood-borne nutrients. Tissue ischemia and related cardiovascular anomalies result in life-threatening complications during childhood, adolescence, and early adulthood. Later the condition causes wrinkled skin. Children with progeria die of heart disease at an average age of thirteen years, with a range of about eight to twenty-one years. At least 90 percent of patients die from complications such as heart attacks or strokes, diseases mostly associated with old age, but their mental development is not affected.

The development of symptoms is comparable to aging, but at a rate six to eight times faster than normal, and certain age-related conditions do not occur. Specifically, patients show no predisposition for neurodegeneration or cancer. They also do not develop "wear and tear" conditions commonly associated with aging, like cataracts and osteoarthritis. Approximately a hundred cases have been formally identified in medical history, but no one knows the real number of current cases. Two families in which more than one child had the disease have been identified. The first was a family in India, who were the subject of a 2005 Bodyshock documentary titled *The Eighty-Year-Old Children*. In 2006 a family in Belgium, who already had one child diagnosed with progeria, were informed that their second child also had the disease.

Cellular and molecular mechanisms involved in progeria are beginning to emerge. A 2003 report in *Nature* said that progeria might be a new trait that has not resulted from other known diseases. According to this theory, progeria develops during cell division in a newly conceived child or in the gametes of one of the parents. This leads to mutations in one of the major architectural proteins of the cell nucleus. Affected nuclei have an architecture that is markedly different from that normally found in healthy nuclei. The mutation occurs in a gene on chromosome number one that leads to the synthesis of new proteins. The new proteins are found near the edge of the nucleus, and they help organize nuclear processes such as the synthesis of RNA and DNA. In progeria the new proteins are mutated, causing the nuclear lesions. The disease can be confirmed through genetic tests, and unlike most other accelerated aging diseases, progeria is not caused by defective DNA repair. Treatment focuses on reducing complications such as cardiovascular disease, and patients have benefited from diets high in calories. Treatment with growth hormone has also been attempted, but no therapy has proved permanently effective; thus there is no known cure for progeria. This leaves it to future research to provide relief for patients and their families who suffer from the disease.

Anxiety and Premature Aging

Anxiety in childhood is associated with problems of emotional, mental, and physical health later in life. Collectively, these problems also lead to premature aging in children. Finding the cause has focused on important physiological systems, including the autonomic nervous system (both its sympathetic and parasympathetic divisions), the hypothalamic-pituitary-adrenal axis (that is, the structural and physiological relations among these three important regulatory organs), the immune system, and genes and chromosomes. These and related investigations have led to important insights about the systemic effects of anxiety and stress in childhood. But the questions of how and when childhood anxiety begins to develop remain unanswered.

In the 1960s it was discovered that fibroblast cells have a built-in mechanism that limits their replicative capacity (ability to reproduce). In the 1970s investigators suggested that telomeres (protein-DNA complexes located at the ends of chromosomes that help determine the number of times a cell will divide and replicate itself) are lost with each replication until a certain minimum is reached (called the Hayflick limit), at which point the cell cycle stops and the cell enters a state of cellular aging. Subsequent research confirmed that telomeres indeed get shorter with each cell division. This established the use of telomeres as molecular clocks for investigating the aging of cells. The advent of efficient laboratory techniques for measuring the length of telomeres has enabled science and medicine to identify risk factors that predict disease. The list of predictable diseases is growing and includes smoking, obesity, psychiatric disorders, and psychosocial anxiety. It has thus been suggested that the length of telomeres is a useful marker for biological aging ("wear and tear") rather than a clock for chronological longevity.

Several recent studies have examined the possible association between childhood anxiety and the length of telomeres. Most of these reports were obtained from adults who recalled cases of anxiety as children growing up (one study of telomeres in kindergarteners is discussed in chapter 3). Results from such anxious children (now adults) were compared with adults, who as children, grew up without experiencing similar anxiety. Telomeres were shorter in the adults who experienced anxiety as children. However, such reports are problematic, in part because longitudinal studies show that the lengths of telomeres are highly variable across different age groups. Reports of adults who experienced anxiety as children are also problematic, because there is an inverse correlation between the lengths of telomeres under baseline conditions and subsequent shortening of telomeres. Also, in some individuals telomeres can lengthen over time. Thus, recent findings indicate that the temporal process of shortening of telomeres is more complex than initially assumed, and that repeated measures, not just one measurement of telomere length at one point in time, are needed to determine if telomeres are shorter in people who have experienced anxiety.

In one study of children, institutional care was associated with shorter telomeres in middle childhood. In another study, investigators set out to determine the influence of bullying on the length of telomeres in victims. They defined bullying in this way: "Someone is being bullied when another child: (1) says mean and hurtful things, makes fun of or calls a person mean and hurtful names; (2) completely ignores or excludes someone from their group of friends or leaves them out of things on purpose; (3) hits, kicks, or shoves a person, or locks them in a room; (4) tells lies or spreads rumors about them; and (5) does other hurtful things like these." The investigators said when it is difficult or impossible for the victim to avoid or prevent the attacks and they occur often, bullying is taking place. When these things are done in a friendly or playful manner, it is not bullying. The study's results provided evidence that anxiety-related accelerated erosion of telomeres can be observed even in early childhood.

Coming of Age Politically

In the United States there are age restrictions of which many of Americans are not aware (tables 1–2 and 1–3). Currently, at age eighteen a person is considered sensible and responsible enough to join the military to kill or be killed for the causes of freedom and democracy. But before 1971 Americans younger than twenty-one could not vote. The case for lowering the voting age to eighteen was made by young Americans on college campuses and elsewhere beginning in the late 1960s, during the Vietnam War (circa 1962–1973). They got organized when former high-school classmates who

TABLE 1-2

Legal Restrictions on Americans by Age

Age (years)	Restriction
18	Minimum age to join the military, vote in public elections, be treated as an adult in a court of law, and buy tobacco products and lottery tickets
21	Minimum age to buy alcohol
25	Minimum age to become a US representative.
30	Minimum age to become a US senator
35	Minimum age to become US president or vice president

TABLE 1-3

Citizenship Class of Americans by Age

Age (years)	Class
0–under 18	Minor or child. No direct political power and limited rights.
18–under 21	Fifth class. Limited adult, with voting rights but cannot hold any upper political offices.
21–under 25	Fourth class. Full adult, but still cannot hold any upper political offices.
25–under 30	Third class. Full adult, can hold limited political offices.
30–under 35	Second class. Full adult, can hold more, but not all, political offices.
35 and over	First class. Full adult who can hold any political office.

had never been eligible to vote began dying in Southeast Asia. Paradoxically, at the same time eighteen-year-olds were legally considered to be adults. They could not only be drafted, but were responsible for their own actions and a court of law could sentence them to prison or even to be executed.

To some people these seemed like double standards. Activists argued that if a person is an adult in a court of law or according to the military, then there is no logical reason to discriminate against that person in other ways, such as preventing him or her from voting. Some also argued that an

adult of any age should be allowed to hold any political office. If a demo-
cratic population voted an eighteen-year-old into public office, then that
population deemed the person qualified and mature enough for the position. In other words, anyone who is old enough to vote is also old enough
to be voted into office. Proponents of lowering the voting age to eighteen
argued that there is no need for an arbitrary age limit for holding a political office (for example, thirty to be a senator and thirty-five to be president). They opposed stratifying adults by age and political rights and
concluded that a person is either mature enough to be an adult, with all
the accompanying risks and benefits, or is a child who needs supervision
and guidance from an adult.

I have been teaching and doing research with students in their early to
mid twenties for nearly forty years. Each semester one of my lecture
courses is taken by 425 juniors, seniors, and graduate students. My teaching laboratory course enrolls 170 similar students. In addition, I teach
much smaller courses. At the end of some semesters I see one or more of
my students with their parents in my office. The parent is there to support
the student in arguing that it is unfair that the student earned a D or F in
my class.

Each year I also have to register my vehicles to park legally on university campuses. I can do this online, but I choose to stand in line instead.
Students with their parents register their vehicles, too. The student often
seems totally disconnected from the task at hand and is preoccupied with
playing a video game on a smart phone or other device. The parent (usually the father) tries to stand inconspicuously in a separate location. When
the student arrives at the cashier's window, the father steps in, questions
the cashier (usually delaying the progress of the line), and then pays for
and receives the necessary decals, hangtags, and so on. I assume that such
parents consider their children incapable of registering a car. The students' disengaged behavior with their video games provides supporting
evidence of this. I wonder if such students are ready to enroll in a university, cast a vote, or go to war. I also wonder how long such parents will
enable their children's immature behavior. Is the twenty-one-year-old student who comes with her parent to my office a child or an adult? Is there
an emerging need for additional stages in how we define adults and children? Perhaps those who according to age are considered legal adults but

according to emotional or social development and behavior have not yet left childhood should be considered chidults or adilds.

Diet and Aging

One problem for the professional investigator of aging is there are no broadly accepted biological markers that can be used to determine the rate of aging. The structural changes (in the way cells, tissues, and organs look) and the functional ones (in the way cells, tissues, and organs work) that occur with time in most adults are not standardized. Another problem is the lack of longitudinal or longevity data. Most people who study aging begin their work after accumulating the necessary credentials, such as PhD or MD degrees. By the time they begin their independent studies, they might be thirty-five years old. These investigators will retire in another twenty-five to thirty-five years—that is, at an age (sixty to seventy years) considerably younger than those they were studying (seventy-five to a hundred years). Therefore, much of the information that could have been collected in the aging subjects is lost during their remaining one to three decades of life. Finding a solution to this problem has been given little attention.

The data show that loss of weight terminating in death commonly occurs in the elderly and is a feature of a geriatric syndrome called failure to thrive. Although in some of the aged the loss in weight is due to disease, in most cases the cause is unknown. My father and my father-in-law died about seven years apart. Observing them in their last years and months was a lesson in living. My father always had a hearty appetite (but was not overweight) and appeared to gain weight during his last years. My father-in-law, on the other hand, was a finicky eater (despite having an excellent cook and baker as a wife); he too was not overweight. In his last years and months he appeared to lose his appetite and considerable weight.

Animal studies have been helpful in trying to understand the relationship between body weight and the aging process. Most rats that live to old ages (two to three and a half years) also exhibit a terminal loss in body weight. Investigators have found the loss of weight in rats to be associated with a decrease in food intake. This, in turn, is related to the consumption of smaller meals eaten in shorter periods of time, rather than to a decreased number of daily meals. Investigators hypothesize that predeath loss of weight associated with aging is caused by a disruption of hormonal balance, particularly in regions of the brain thought to control hunger and food intake (including the hypothalamus, the pituitary, and their interactions). The neurochemical changes in the brain (for example, in the rates of production, release, storage, and action of chemicals and hormones) result in deregulation of food intake relative to the animal's needs for energy.

Since the mid-1970s investigators have carried out life-span studies on male rats. Findings reveal that loss of weight during aging is not always associated with decreased intake of food. Detailed data on body weight, food intake throughout the life span, and pathological lesions at the time of spontaneous death became available in the 1980s and early 1990s. One study involved a group of rats that had free access to food and water, and another group of rats whose consumption of food (but not water) was restricted—starting when they were about six weeks old—to 60 percent of the daily intake of the first group of rats. The underfed rats were healthier and lived longer than their counterparts with free access to food. This regimen, which investigators refer to as dietary or calorie restriction, is known to markedly slow the rate of aging in laboratory rodents.

In April 2012 in San Diego, I attended an annual meeting called Experimental Biology. I was excited about hearing a keynote address by David Sabatini. The lecture hall was packed with an estimated fifteen hundred attendees; it was standing room only. Sabatini was honored by the American Society for Biochemistry and Molecular Biology as the inaugural recipient of its Earl and Thressa Stadtman Scholar Award. Sabatini received the award for his work in identifying the mTOR pathway. Mammalian target of rapamycin (mTOR) is a major protein regulator of mammalian cell growth and a central component of pathways relating to metabolism and aging. Sabatini gave us his views of how mTOR is able to sense cellular changes in the availability of oxygen, energy (related to food intake), and intrinsically produced growth factors, and how these relate to tissue function and survival. He showed us some of the most recent research data, which illustrated that by reducing the daily intake of calories, both the health and longevity of experimental animals and humans increases.

Sabatini's message that day was simple and clear: eat less and be healthier. After his presentation the discussion focused, in part, on people who adhere to the practice of reducing their intake of calories by 20–40 percent of the recommended daily allowance of 2,000 calories for adults. In most of the cases studied to date, their health improves. Definitive determination of the effects of restricting calories on longevity in such people will have to wait several more decades for the data to be collected.

Although questions about longevity and human health have been asked since the beginning of time, investigators have only been collecting and reporting data since the 1930s. And most of those results have been obtained in experimental animals. For example, of the more than forty genetic strains of mice being studied, about half live longer when calories are restricted. But just as many had shorter lives than they would have had on a normal diet without a restriction in calories. Similarly, in August 2012, a long-running experiment on monkeys at the National Institute on Aging concluded that after twenty-five years monkeys whose calories were restricted showed no aging advantage. Still, in many animal species studied to date, including invertebrates, restricting the daily intake of calories by 20–60 percent increases longevity and health. Studies in humans have begun only in recent decades, but early results—including those reported by investigators like David Sabatini and Luigi Fontana—are most encouraging. However, it appears that the jury is still out on questions of diet, health, and longevity.

Groups such as the Calorie Restriction Society International follow serious diet-related health codes. Seventh Day Adventists and Mormons (members of the Church of Jesus Christ of Latter-Day Saints) do, too. James Enstrom, a non-Mormon epidemiologist at the University of California, Los Angeles, has been studying Mormons in Southern California for several decades. He reports that in all causes of disease and death, Mormons are healthier than the general population and live eight to ten years longer. Actively practicing Mormons adhere to a diet and health code they call the Word of Wisdom. This code identifies things that people should and should not take into their bodies. According to the Word of Wisdom, things that should not be consumed include tobacco, alcohol, and hot drinks (interpreted to mean coffee, tea, and related products). Mormons are also encouraged to eat meat sparingly. Things the Word of Wisdom encourages people to consume include a generous supply of fruits and vegetables that are in season (or preserved for consumption during other seasons) and wheat (whole or cracked) and wheat products. This health code was adopted by the church around 1838–1851.

In addition to these dietary and nutritional guidelines, actively practicing Mormons subscribe to a regimen of physical fitness, adequate sleep and rest, and a lifetime of learning (secular and doctrinal or theological). Mormons I have observed who do these things are some of the happiest, most well-adjusted people I know. And there are other groups and data to support the notion that using wisdom in one's eating practices is good for one's health. These include the dietary practices of Orthodox Jews and the restricted consumption of animal products by Hindus, vegetarians, vegans, and the like.

Theories of Aging

The age of an individual usually refers to the length of time he or she has lived. This is as applicable to invertebrates (such as a fruit fly) and other vertebrate animals (like a dog or cat) as it is to humans. Investigators as well as the general public usually think of aging as becoming less functional. You might look at a man and say he looks old for his age. This to you would mean that the processes of aging seem to be occurring rapidly in that individual. If the person looked young for his age, the opposite would be true. I have known fit and unfit people during most of my life. When I question fit people about how they feel, it is not uncommon to hear exclamations such as, "I feel twenty years younger than I am!" This means that they feel physiologically less aged than their actual chronological age. Rarely do I hear similar comments from the unfit.

The processes of physiological aging are easily measurable in family members, other loved ones, neighbors, and co-workers. In 2012 my dentist retired. He had treated me for nearly thirty-six years, and we were more than doctor and patient. We had become friends, and we could observe and talk about the processes of aging in each other. I have missed our association, including seasonal discussions about Rutgers University football and basketball. Like the lines on a football field and their ability to mark a team's progress, biomarkers are chemicals, functions, and structures used by biologists to glean information about living events. For example, if an animal lacks oxygen, the contents and partial pressures of oxygen in that animal's circulating blood (biomarkers) will be reduced. This will lead to lack of tissue oxygenation (hypoxia) and to a poor prognosis if the condition is not quickly reversed. It would be helpful to have a definitive list of physiologically important molecules, functions, and structures to mark the rate of our aging (for example, indicating that we are now at the fifty-yard line). Alas, science and medicine cannot agree on such a list, so there is none. Doesn't this seem odd, especially when one thinks about the wrinkles (lines) on the face of an aging person? Wouldn't it be quite simple to develop a system for rating the quantity and quality of such wrinkles as markers of normal aging? (Distractors like cosmetic facial surgery and Botox injections are topics for other books.)

Unlike the aging of individuals, for about two centuries we have been able to measure the aging of populations. For example, in 1825 a British actuary by the name of Benjamin Gompertz published a report on age-specific death rates in his country. Gompertz defined an age-specific death rate as the fraction of the population entering an interval of age (such as 50–59) that dies during that interval. After young adulthood (ages 20–40), Gompertz found that the age-specific death rate increases exponentially with advancing age. The same is true in human populations other than the British and in animal populations as well. Whether or not disease is a fundamental component of aging is controversial. Gerontologists have coined the phrase "age-associated diseases" as those that do not cause mortality until advanced age. Examples include atherogenic coronary artery disease, stroke, type II diabetes, osteoarthritis and osteoporosis, cataracts, macular degeneration, Alzheimer's disease, and Parkinson's disease. These are either chronic or acute, and they usually result from long-term events (such as atherosclerosis). However, as our society becomes increasingly overweight and obese, what used to be thought of as age-associated disease (for example, type II diabetes) are showing up in childhood and adolescence at an alarming rate. Gerontologists now distinguish between primary and secondary aging. Primary aging refers to intrinsic changes that occur with age and that are unrelated to disease and the environment. Secondary aging includes interactions between primary aging and disease and the environment.

In 1900 about 4 percent of the US population was sixty-five years and older. In 2010 that age group had increased to 13 percent. Between 2000 and 2010 the number of Americans ages forty-five to sixty-four grew 32 percent, to about 82 million. The increased rate of growth in this age group is primarily due to the aging of the baby boomers (who were born between 1946 and 1963, so some investigators say the baby boomer generation turned sixty-six in January 2012). The population ages sixty-five and older also grew faster than most younger groups, at a rate of 15 percent—reaching 40 million people. For those under eighteen and between the ages of eighteen and forty-four, growth rates were much slower. Between 2000 and 2010, the number of people under eighteen grew 2.6 percent, to 74 million, or 24 percent of the total population. The population ages eighteen to forty-four grew even more slowly, at a rate of less than 1 percent. These people now number 113 million, or 37 percent of the population.

According to some authorities, this trend in the structure of the aging US population is projected to continue. The increase in age structure in the United States during the twentieth century had very little to do with improved health and medicine. Rather, it was caused by a marked decline in the rate of new births. This "repropause" (a pause in reproduction, like menopause or andropause, a phenomenon in men that is similar to menopause in women) single-handedly led the elderly to become an increasingly larger fraction of the growing US population. However, the rate of decline in births in the United States cannot drop much lower than it is at present. Therefore, future changes in the age structure will have more to do with changes in our health and longevity.

One other statistic in US demographics is noteworthy. As of May 2012, and for the first time in US history, the birth rates of minority groups surpassed that of Caucasians of European descent. In other words, Black, Hispanic, Asian, and other minority groups are now producing the majority of newborns in the United States. Minority populations still have less access to affordable health insurance and quality health care than Whites do. If this continues, the socioeconomic burden of the aging population will increase.

Humor and Aging

As serious as aging and health are, everyone has their favorite humorous anecdotes and stories about aging. This is one of mine: There were two elderly people, John and Helen, who lived in a suburban mobile home park. He was a widower, she was a widow, and they had known each other for a number of years. One evening at a community supper, the two found themselves seated across from each other. As the evening progressed, John glanced admiringly at Helen several times, and he finally gathered his courage to ask, "Helen, will you marry me?" After about five seconds of careful consideration, Helen answered, "Yes. Yes, I will." The meal ended, and with a few more pleasant exchanges they went their respective ways. Next morning John was troubled. Did Helen say yes or no? He couldn't remember. In humiliation he went to the telephone and called Helen. He explained that he didn't remember things as well as he used to. Then he reviewed the enjoyable previous evening. As he gained a little more courage, John inquired gingerly, "Helen, when I asked if you would marry me, did you say yes or no?" John was delighted to hear Helen say, "Why, I said, yes, yes I will, and I meant it with all my heart." Then she continued, "I am so glad that you called, John, because I couldn't remember for the life of me who had asked."

Several of my retired colleagues and I meet once each semester for lunch. This allows me to learn about retirement from them, and for us all to catch up on recent events inside and outside the university. At one recent lunch the topic turned to signs of aging in all of us. One man mentioned that the names of people, even those who are most familiar to him, don't come as easily as they did a few years ago. Another mentioned his inability to perform manual labor for more than three or four hours now, compared to the six or eight he used to spend on Saturdays a few years ago. One colleague told us of pouring a cup of coffee on his cold breakfast cereal, which prompted another to tell of returning the jug of milk to the cupboard. Some of these incidents were funny, and most of them had to do with short-term memory.

A few years before my father's death, my wife and I were visiting my parents and her aunt and uncle. Both of the older men were World War II veterans, and my father was also a veteran of the Korean War. The men were sharing war stories. Uncle Royal asked my father how old he was. When Uncle Royal learned that he was a few years older than my father, he said, "Hell, you're just a youngster." I know this didn't sit well with my dad, but the conversation continued and soon the women joined in. Aunt Rhea made a couple of comments about others who had served in the wars. When it came my dad's turn to talk again, his tongue got twisted (too many names beginning with the letter R). He had also just met the uncle and aunt for the first time. Not remembering who was who, he tried to address Royal but could only stammer until he blurted out "Ralph." This caught me off-guard, and I burst out laughing. Both my dad and I had known several Ralphs in our small mountain community in Wyoming. The name conjured up funny memories (including television's Jackie Gleason as Ralph the bus driver). My outburst stimulated a similar laugh from my wife. Then the older women joined in, and soon we were all enjoying a memorable moment of war, words, and laughter. That is a good memory of my deceased dad.

During the spring of 1985, I was completing a sabbatical at the Texas College of Osteopathic Medicine in Fort Worth (now North Texas State University Health Sciences Center). After eating my lunch on the spacious lawn adjacent to the Fort Worth Public Library, I went inside. Wandering through the library, I couldn't help notice the feet of someone wearing white socks and no shoes. I took a closer look. There was an old man thumbing through the card catalogue. He noticed me, and I smiled and said hello. I judged him to be in his mid-eighties. My hello encouraged a short conversation, after which we exchanged names (his was Bill), shook hands, and went our separate ways. A few days later I returned to the library, found Bill there again, and had another brief talk with him. This experience was repeated several times over the next few weeks.

After we had gotten to know each other, Bill asked, "Would you like to come to my house for lunch some time?" I said yes and thanked him for his kind offer. When I arrived, he made peanut butter and jelly sandwiches and poured a couple of glasses of milk, and we sat down to eat. During the conversation Bill said, "You know, I have never given a child or grandchild a piggyback ride." I listened, reflecting on the countless times I had done that with my own children. We sat silent for several seconds, and then Bill asked, "Can I give you a piggyback ride?" My heart sank. I weighed about 180 pounds at the time and was nearly six feet tall. I judged Bill to be no more than five and a half feet tall, and he couldn't have weighed more than 125 pounds.

I said, "Bill, how about starting with a horsyback ride first?" He agreed and we went through the motions. By the end of the ride my much-younger knees and hips were kinked, but Bill was elated and encouraged. He had just given his first horsyback ride. Then he asked excitedly, "Can I give you a piggyback ride now?" I lovingly set the limits (time, distance, location) and complied. Thankfully, Bill did not collapse (during both rides I made my feet reach the floor to support the bulk of my weight). At nearly eighty-five years of age, this man had given his first horsy- and piggyback rides to a stranger. I was happy to momentarily act like the child or grandchild he never had.

During the next few months we continued to meet at the library. On one occasion Bill invited my family and me to have dinner with him. At the time our oldest children were teenagers. They got a roar out of the stories I told about Bill but weren't interested in dinner. Our younger children felt sorry for the old man and wanted to go. We had a wonderful evening. Of all the interpersonal experiences I had that year living among Texans, this one has been the most memorable for me.

Mechanisms of Aging

Cellular and molecular biology has taken front and center stage in recent decades in the life sciences. Therefore, the debate on what causes aging focuses on the way aging affects cells and important biomolecules. There are several schools of thought about the mechanisms involved. The theories include: (1) oxidative stress and its influences on large, biologically important molecules; (2) damage to cellular organelles such as the energy factories or mitochondria; (3) damage to DNA; (4) inadequate cellular repair processes; and (5) dysfunction in the physiological regulation of the number of cells.

While revising this chapter in July 2013, I attended the 37th Congress of the International Union of Physiological Sciences in Birmingham, England. One of the symposia focused on aging cells in the cardiovascular system. One speaker showed evidence that eliminating aged cells in mice reduces the characteristics of aging in that species. Another talked about the role of a family of proteins called sirtuins. He said that eliminating sirtuin-6 (the most studied among these proteins) induces the characteristics of aging, impairs the formation of capillaries (which reduces blood flow) and promotes damage to DNA and telomeres. Thus, if diminished sirtuin-6 is one of the causes of aging, then replenishing sirtuin-6 should attenuate the effects of aging. Doubtless, there will be more investigation of these and related topics in years to come.

Loss of mass of tissue (including sarcopenia, or the loss of muscle mass, muscle strength, and muscle endurance) is a characteristic of aging. One gram of tissue from a small mammal (such as a mouse) has a higher resting metabolic rate than one gram of tissue from a larger mammal (such as a horse). The life cycle of smaller animals is correspondingly shorter than that of large animals. However, when the resting metabolic rate is normalized for either the age or weight of the animal, both small and large animals expend a similar amount of energy during their lifetimes. Because of this, some investigators at the beginning of the twentieth century proposed that animals have a finite amount of "vital principle" that they deplete at the rate of energy expenditure. Subsequent research failed to support this conclusion about aging but helped begin characterizing the aging phenotype (dubbed the "rate of living" theory of aging). Table 1–4 presents a summary of some of the effects of aging on major mammalian organ systems.

The physiology of reactive oxygen species (ROS) has been at the center of the aging debate for the last few decades. Reactive oxygen species, also called oxidants, include compounds such as hydrogen peroxide (H_2O_2), hydroxyl radical ($^{\bullet}OH$), superoxide anion (O_2^-) and peroxynitrite ($ONOO^-$). These are unstable compounds that react with target molecules to capture their electrons, thus making the target molecules unstable. ROS—particularly $^{\bullet}OH$ and $ONOO^-$, the most reactive of them all—have the ability to damage important biological molecules such as proteins, lipids, DNA, and RNA, all four of which are essential building blocks for cells and their subcellular organelles. Thus, they have important effects on cellular functions. Proteins and lipids constitute the fabric of cell membranes. Membrane-bound proteins serve as channels, pores, pumps, and transporters. As such, they help regulate the internal and external environments of the cell. They allow the passage of water, move small charged chemicals and molecules into and out of the cells, and are essential for life.

Another class of oxidants are the reactive nitrogen species. In addition, the very important signaling molecule, nitric oxide (NO), is a highly reactive molecule. Despite the harm that ROS and other chemicals can

TABLE 1-4

A Summary of Aging Effects in Major Mammalian Organ Systems

System	Effect
Nervous	Decrease in sensory functions (touch, hearing, vision), slowing of both reaction time and central processing
Endocrine	Decrease in function of all organs (pituitary, pancreas, adrenals, thyroid, etc.), resistance to insulin and impaired glucose tolerance, impairment of diurnal or circadian rhythms
Reproductive	Perimenopause and menopause in women, erectile dysfunction and andropause in men
Urinary	Decline in filtration (begins by age thirty in some people but is not inevitable), tubular reuptake decreases, incontinence, BPH[a]
Gastrointestinal	Loss of muscle in sphincters, with resulting problems in swallowing and release of stool
Musculoskeletal	Loss of height and lean body mass; gain and redistribution of body fat; increasing weakness, brittleness, and stiffness in tissues
Cardiovascular	Hardening of vessels, especially arteries; weakened cardiac function; elevated blood pressure
Respiratory	Weakening of muscles of respiration (diaphragm, intercostals), decreasing lung volume and capacity
Skin	Loss of moisture, wrinkles, thinning epidermis, decreased melanocytes (which give the skin color), reduced photoprotection

[a]BPH (benign prostate hyperplasia, or enlargement of the prostate) can affect both the renal (urinary) and reproductive systems.

cause, they also perform important physiological and biochemical functions. They play essential roles in the destruction of bacteria and other pathogens in phagocytic cells (cells that destroy things that are foreign to the body). They also contribute to the formation of thyroid hormones by altering the metabolism of iodide anions. Ionizing radiation can produce ROS, but their most important source is the electron transport chain inside the mitochondria—in other words, mitochondria produce ROS.

Thus, they are an active ingredient in cellular metabolism, use of oxygen, and production of waste products such as carbon dioxide.

Less than 1 percent of the oxygen we consume each day is used by the mitochondria to generate ROS. However, in the absence of protective antioxidant systems even that amount would be lethal to cells and tissues. Fortunately, we have built-in antioxidant systems. The most well characterized and thoroughly investigated are enzymes, including catalase, glutathione peroxidase, and superoxide dismutase (the names of most enzymes end in the suffix *ase*). These are endogenous systems (produced by our bodies). There are also exogenous antioxidant systems (not produced by the body), such as the low-molecular-weight vitamins A, C, and E, as well as acetaminophen and other over-the-counter products. Moreover, according to the US Department of Agriculture and its Healthy People 2010 initiative, the grains and vegetables we should all be eating for improved health are full of antioxidants, including the vitamins just mentioned. Doubtless there are other antioxidants in these food products that are as yet undiscovered. Fruits are another source of antioxidants. There is ample evidence that people who consume these food products throughout their lives age more successfully than nonconsumers. Finally, I refer the more curious advanced reader to some of my research highlighting the antioxidant, protective actions of acetaminophen in the hearts and brains of experimental animals.

Mitochondria are the major source of production of ROS, so it should not be surprising that they are also one of the main targets of ROS. Mitochondria produce DNA (mitochondrial DNA, or mtDNA), and damage to mtDNA increases greatly with age because cellular mechanisms are not in place to prevent it (unlike the case with nuclear DNA). Damage to mtDNA impairs the synthesis and therefore reduces the availability of adenosine triphosphate (ATP, an important source of energy for cellular function). Damage to both nuclear and mitochondrial DNA can be caused by dangerous chemicals and the environment (for example, radiation). Cells can repair much of the damage, so there is a balance between damage and repair. The accumulation of damaged DNA can interfere with many vital cellular functions, including the cell's ability to replicate itself (see the discussion of progeria and premature aging above). Collectively, these processes have been referred to as the "mitochondrial/DNA damage theory of aging." Mitochondria are also the major site of synthesis of ATP.

The above mechanisms emphasize enzymatic reactions between good and bad chemicals in living tissues. There are other nonenzymatic reactions that involve simple sugars and their interactions with proteins to form advanced glycation endproducts, or AGEs. The familiar brown hue in a potato that has been cut up and boiled results from these and additional reactions that produce coloring compounds in the cells. The formation of AGEs is especially important with long-lived proteins and might be involved in the long-term complications of diabetes. Similarities between the appearance of an aging individual and someone with diabetes have led scientists to develop the "glycation hypothesis of aging." This is just one of the reasons for the medical concerns with elevated blood glucose (for example, Mayor Michael Bloomberg's attempts to regulate large, sugar-laden drinks in New York City, circa 2012–13). For example, AGEs can interact with proteins of the eye and thereby contribute to opacity, macular degeneration, and other visual impairments.

According to classic mammalian physiology, there are a small handful of major organ systems in humans. They include: (1) the brain and spinal cord (central nervous system); (2) the adrenal and other endocrine glands (endocrine system); (3) the immune system; (4) the female and male internal and external genitalia (reproductive system); (5) the kidneys, bladder, and ureters or urethra (renal or urinary system); (6) the stomach, gut, and accessory tissues (gastrointestinal system); (7) the musculoskeletal system; (8) the heart and blood vessels (cardiovascular system); and (9) the lungs and respiratory passages (respiratory system). The changes described above that take place at the cellular and molecular levels also affect whole organs and the systems they belong to. In our research laboratory, my colleagues and I investigate the mammalian cardiovascular system. Among other things, we have studied the regulation of coronary blood flow and the rhythmicity of the cardiac cycle. We have done this in states of good physiological health and in states of disease and injury. In recent years we have included the brain in our experiments.

In our research on hearts and brains, we have found that acetaminophen can protect mitochondrial structure and function during cellular injury. Acetaminophen is a phenol and, as such, has important antioxidant properties. For one thing, the drug helps keep the double-walled mitochondrial membrane structure intact during periods of ischemia and reperfusion injury. This is important because essential regulatory proteins span the parallel outer and inner mitochondrial membranes and thus determine the passage of chemicals between them. One of these is the so-called proton pump. It helps maintain the level of acidity or alkalinity inside the mitochondria, which is important to their function and survival. We do not yet know if these animal-based results are applicable to humans, but we are moving toward experimentation with humans.

Sadly, many people show marked deterioration in all major organ systems early in the aging process, and others who show decay in at least some systems. Although the aging process is similar in both genders, important differences exist. No one questions the existence of aging-related menopause in women, but there is much debate and considerable doubt about the existence of what is called andropause in aging men. Not until 2013 did I become aware of advertisements for hormone replacement therapy in men (for reduced circulating concentrations of testosterone, a condition known as low-T). Repropause, or the marked reduction in birth rates in industrialized nations in the past few decades, is the well-known and main cause of aging of the populations of all those nations.

In summary, aging affects people differently. A few humans show minimal signs of deterioration with age. They are said to have undergone "successful aging." According to the Bible, Moses was one such person: "And Moses was an hundred and twenty years old when he died: his eye was not dim nor his natural force abated" (Deuteronomy 34:7). Just before the Flood, God told Noah (who was then about 600 years old, according to Genesis 7:6) that at some future point after the Flood, the span of human life would be 120 years (Genesis 6:3). We are living in that future. As I've already mentioned, there are supercentenarians today, those who live to be 110–120 years old. The cover of the May 2013 issue of *National Geographic* magazine displays the photo of an infant, with a legend that declares: "This baby will live to be 120." The accompanying article by Stephen S. Hall tries to support the notion that we can all live to that age.

So, here's to healthy aging. As you age, may you be wise enough to stop bad habits, eat a nutritious diet, exercise regularly, and pay more attention to the children than to the animals.

2

The Aging Nervous System

GYMNAST: Can you teach me to do the splits?
GYMNASTICS INSTRUCTOR: How flexible are you?
GYMNAST: Well, I can't come in on Thursdays.

Studies conducted during the past forty years have shown that a good, hearty laugh—as opposed to loud, boisterous laughter—can relieve tension and stress, strengthen the immune system, and reduce the risk of heart attack and stroke. Healthy laughter and humor can be a tonic for the brain, as well. The next time you hear a joke, whether you get it or not, let yourself go. Laughter is good for the brain, the nervous systems, and you.

Laughter is partially coordinated by the central nervous system, which consists of the brain and spinal cord. The central nervous system is only one component of the complete nervous system of humans. Other components include the somatic (body) or peripheral nervous system, the autonomic nervous system, and the enteric nervous system. The somatic system makes our limbs and other peripheral body parts work, the autonomic system controls involuntary parts and functions such as the endocrine system and heart and respiratory rates, and the enteric system operates our digestive tract (controlling its secretions, movements, digestion, and absorption). The somatic nervous system includes nerve tracts that project from the spinal cord to the fingers and toes, skin and hair, and other peripheral sites, as well as tracts that carry sensory information from the periphery to the spinal cord and brain. The autonomic nervous system is mainly an efferent, motor nervous system. It has also been called the involuntary or vegetative nervous system. Cell bodies in its nerve tracts originate in the thoracic and lumbar regions of the spinal cord (the sympathetic nervous system) and inside the cranium and the sacral spinal cord (the parasympathetic nervous system). The sensory input that this nervous system receives is the same as that derived from the peripheral nervous system (in other words, the autonomic is not a sensory nervous system). Finally, the enteric nervous system, which some people call the little brain, is confined to the walls of the gastrointestinal tract. It has both sensory and motor components and is concerned primarily with gastrointestinal functions.

The basic units involved in the function and structure of the human nervous system include neurons, glial cells (or glia), oligodendrocytes, and others (such as pyramidal cells and basket cells). Neurons function primarily as communication cables, while glia (including astrocytes) provide biochemical support to vascular endothelial cells in the blood-brain barrier, nutritional support for the nervous tissue, maintenance of extracellular ion balance, and repair and remodeling processes in the brain and spinal cord following traumatic injuries. Astrocytes are the most abundant cell in the human brain. Oligodendrocytes play supportive roles for neurons, including insulating the axons of the central nervous system, a function similar to that of the Schwann cells in the peripheral nervous system. The basic neuron consists of a cell body (or soma) where the nucleus and other subcellular organelles reside, a longer extension that projects from the soma to other neurons or cells and is called the axon, and shorter projections from the soma called dendrites. Dendrites serve as docking stations for adjacent neurons. Of course, there are other elements and finer details, but what I have said here will suffice for the following discussion of the aging nervous system.

The Aging Cerebral Cortex

By 2030 nearly one in five US residents is expected to be sixty-five or older. This age group is projected to increase from about 39 million in 2010 to 88 million in 2050. In Western cultures, this age group has been and will continue to be stereotyped negatively—as lonely, crotchety, sluggish, feeble, frequently hospitalized, and cognitively impaired. These negative stereotypes often have the unfortunate effect of perpetuating the belief that cognitive decline is normal and inevitable. Stereotypes of aging are also present in science. For example, in human neuroscience, the aged brain has historically been stereotyped as brittle and nonconforming, with little room for new growth. Happily, more recent investigations have begun to break down these stereotypes. New findings suggest that the aging brain is both plastic and responsive. Fortunately, these break-throughs challenge the definition of normal aging and the amount of brain deterioration or cognitive decline that should be deemed acceptable or normal.

Paul Leath, a physicist, was associate provost for the sciences at Rutgers University in the 1980s. I see him occasionally as I sit on a bench on the Busch Campus of Rutgers and watch people passing by. He is almost always surrounded by two or more young people. His walking pace matches theirs, and he seems as familiar with them as they are with him. I assume these younger folks are his postdocs, graduate students, and other members of his laboratory or the Physics Department. I also assume that he surrounds himself with young people, in part, as an anti-aging strategy. Leath is a smart man. And what he's doing is a good thing for Rutgers University and its oral history project. People like Leath have extensive memories of the recent history of institutions (the past forty to fifty years) and are invaluable resources for documenting such histories. You can go online and learn about research in physics and astronomy at Rutgers by reading recent interviews with Leath.

With advanced age comes a decline in sensorimotor control and func-tioning. The deteriorations in fine motor control, gait, and balance affect the ability of older adults to perform activities of daily living and to main-tain their independence. The causes of such deficits are multifactorial, with impairment of the central nervous system and changes in sensory receptors, muscles, and peripheral nerves playing major roles. Aging is also accompanied by marked changes in muscle strength and motor control. Many of these changes result from an overwhelming number of structural complications in the motor cortex, which controls most of the body's movements.

Examinations of humans who died without neurological disease reveal that individuals over sixty-five exhibit about a 43 percent reduction in the size of cell bodies in neurons in the premotor cortex, compared to adults younger than forty-five. These observations have been corroborated in living humans with high-resolution structural magnetic resonance imaging (MRI). In one investigation, researchers obtained images from 106 individuals without dementia who were eighteen to ninety-three years old. Atrophy of the cortex occurred by middle age and was most severe nearest the primary motor cortex. In addition, the mass of white matter and the length of myelinated neurons decreased by about 45 percent between ages eighteen and ninety-three. Other age-related changes in the motor cortex included reduced excitability of neurons, reduced size and number of motor units (an individual motor nerve and all the muscle fibers it innervates), and altered discharge properties of motor units.

During fetal development in rhesus monkeys, neurons in the motor cortex appear earlier than neurons in other cortical regions, including the hippocampus. In cats the lateral regions of the motor cortex develop before the medial subdivision. However, the development order of neurons cannot account for the selective vulnerability of neurons in some layers of this organ (the "first in, first out" hypothesis). If the earliest neurons to develop were those most susceptible to aging, then the deep neurons in deeper layers of the motor cortex would be most vulnerable, since the cortex forms in an inside-out pattern.

Among important structural and physiological changes, aging of the human brain is associated with molecular changes that underlie alterations in intelligence, learning, memory, and mood. Typical aging can also constrain the onset of neurological diseases that range from late-onset neurodegeneration such as Alzheimer's and Parkinson's diseases to early-onset psychiatric conditions such as bipolar disorder and schizophrenia. The molecular mechanisms and genetic underpinnings of age-related changes in the brain are underinvestigated. And although they overlap somewhat with peripheral changes, many are unique to the brain, whose cells mostly do not divide. Hence, understanding the aging brain and identifying associated markers and mechanisms will have profound consequences for the prevention and treatment of age-related impairments and diseases.

Physiological aging-related decreases in neurological functioning (that is, those observed in the absence of brain-related diseases) have been extensively studied, with robust and consistent results. For example, a meta-analysis of cross-sectional and longitudinal data sets demonstrated a 40–60 percent decline in cognitive speed at age eighty compared to age twenty in adults without dementia. Moreover, psychosomatic activities that rely on processing speed, problem solving, inhibitory function, working memory, long-term memory, and spatial orientation decline with age. Conversely, so-called crystallized abilities—one's personal qualities that relate to knowledge or expertise, such as vocabulary, knowledge of history or world events, general information, implicit memory, understanding of proverbs, and career or occupational skills—do not decline or may even show improvement over the life span. Consistent with this observation is the fact that one's verbal IQ declines only modestly from age twenty to age seventy.

In addition to cognitive and morphological changes in the aging brain, age also affects neurochemistry. Age-induced changes in neurotransmitters and their receptors are probably associated with decreases in both cognitive and motor functions. Impaired neurotransmission is responsible for at least some of the behavioral abnormalities associated with aging. For example, Arvid Carlsson's Nobel Prize–winning work indicated that depletion of the neurotransmitter dopamine underlies the motor deficits in Parkinson's disease. Normal age-related changes have also been observed in the production, storage, and release of other neurotransmitters such as serotonin, acetylcholine, norepinephrine, gamma amino butyric acid, and glutamate, and are also associated with reductions in growth factors in the motor cortex.

Neurogenesis and the Aging Hippocampus

There was much excitement about the detection in the late 1990s of adult neurogenesis in the human central nervous system. Neurogenesis is the ability of the adult nervous system to generate new brain cells. It was predicted that in the near future, neural stem cells could be the basis for cell replacement and regeneration in the diseased brain or for improved cognition during aging.

Neurogenesis is a process mediated by molecular and physiological factors. Specific molecules such as the vascular endothelial growth factor, as well as exposure to a pleasing environment, have been shown to significantly stimulate neurogenesis. In the case of one's environment, my colleague and friend Karl Herrup, an expert on Alzheimer's disease, has recently found that when subjects with Alzheimer's are periodically exposed to simulated Japanese botanical gardens, they do better than when left in their stagnant and unstimulating institutional bedrooms. Moreover, the intensification of voluntary physical activity achieves results similar to enhancing the surrounding environment. In contrast, stress throughout the aging process causes marked declines in the rates of neurogenesis. One of the structures of the nervous system that is intimately involved in emotions and cognition is the hippocampus.

The hippocampus is in a unique position to influence and be influenced by multiple brain areas. For example, it lies in close anatomical proximity to the limbic system and shares connections with that system and adjacent brain structures. Connections also exist between the hippocampus and the amygdala, the cerebral cortex, and sub-cortical tissues. Additional connections come from the dentate gyrus, septal nuclei, raphe nuclei, the hypothalamus, and numerous brainstem structures such as the locus coeruleus. All of these structures and others are involved in physiological regulation, learning, and memory. The great importance of these structures and their connections in humans explains why many studies of cognition and aging have focused on trying to understand hippocampal neurogenesis. A prevailing assumption in the field of adult neurogenesis is that the continuous generation of new neurons in the hippocampus does not only offer the formation of new synapses between neurons, but also provides a cellular flexibility to the central nervous system. This could be especially crucial for memory and learning. Newly generated neurons are particularly excitable and are thought to be more sensitive to incoming input than older neurons.

The hippocampus receives sensory input from the cerebral cortex. This information is processed and then sent back to cortical areas of association. The fundamental importance of the hippocampus in the transition from short-term memory (functional memory/working memory, lasting seconds to minutes) to long-term memory (requiring the transcription of genes and the synthesis of new proteins, lasting minutes to hours or longer) first became evident with patients whose hippocampi (plural of hippocampus) were surgically removed due to otherwise untreatable epilepsy. Following surgery these patients were not able to transfer any new memory into long-term storage (called anterograde amnesia).

One element of episodic memory that is also accessible in rodents is spatial memory (rats navigating a laboratory maze; people navigating a cornfield maze). Aging decreases performance in tasks of spatial navigation across species (humans, subhuman primates, rats, and mice). Aging not only impairs storage of spatial memory, it also reduces one's capacity to encode memory quickly, which might be crucial in coping with sudden and unexpected changes in environments or experiences. Significantly, in addition to spatial learning and memory, a variety of other hippocampus-dependent functions such as fear conditioning and eye-blink conditioning are affected by age and decline over a lifetime. Despite growing recognition that the aged brain retains some capacity for neurogenesis, there is significant evidence for brain atrophy with advancing age. For example, longitudinal studies have reported a 1–2 percent annual atrophy of the hippocampus in adults older than fifty-five years without dementia. Estimated rates of atrophy of 0.5–2.0 percent per year occur in other regions of the brain, including the prefrontal cortex, caudate nucleus, and the cerebellum. Conversely, the primary motor and sensorimotor regions of the cortex seem to be relatively unaffected by age.

Discovering the molecular mechanisms that contribute to loss of brain tissue in late adulthood has become an important objective in recent years. There are multiple explanations, at the cellular or molecular levels, for the atrophy of brain tissue in humans, including increased apoptosis. Apoptosis is the so-called programmed cell death, or the notion that cells are preprogrammed to last for a finite period and that they know when to stop functioning. Other explanations for age-related atrophy of the brain include decreased cell proliferation, degeneration of axons, reductions in the populations of dendrites and the density of spines emerging from them, shrinkage of cell bodies, reduced vascularity and blood supply, and any combination of these. In fact, given the variability in the rates of atrophy across the brain, it is unlikely that any single change in molecules or cellular structures or events could satisfactorily explain the loss of tissue volume with age. Indeed, research in rats and mice suggests that increased rates of cell death are unlikely to explain the atrophy associated with normal aging. This implies that contributions from other factors—for example, the decline of dendritic spines with age—are also important.

Several molecules have attracted considerable interest because of their hypothetical roles in dementias and cellular aging. These include beta amyloid; inflammatory markers such as interleukins-2, -6, and -15; stress hormones like cortisol and deoxycorticosterone; and brain-derived neurotrophic factor. This factor is found in high concentrations in the hippocampus and the cerebral cortex and is critical to the development of memory, neurogenesis, and cell proliferation. Changes in it are associated with age-related loss of memory, depression, and atrophy of the hippocampus.

The Brainstem

Joining the cerebral hemispheres and nearby structures (such as the cerebellum) to the spinal cord is the brainstem. The main components of the mammalian brainstem are the pons and medulla. The pons is above the medulla and adjacent to structures such as the hypothalamus. The medulla lies below the pons and is attached to the cervical segment of the spinal column. Both the pons and the medulla are locations of physiologically important control and regulatory centers in the central nervous system. For example, the cardiovascular and respiratory control centers are found in the medulla. The cardiovascular control centers regulate vasomotor functions such as the degrees of constriction and relaxation of blood vessels. They also control cardiac functions such as heart rate and rhythmicity. The respiratory control centers regulate frequencies of ventilation and the volumes of air that enter and exit the lungs during each respiratory cycle. Collectively, these control centers determine the general homeostasis of the cardiovascular and respiratory systems, including important physiological variables such as blood pressure, heart rate, respiratory rhythmicity, and the matching of blood flow (perfusion) and air flow (ventilation), known as the ventilation-to-perfusion ratio. Among other regulatory sites found in the pons is the micturition center. Working with higher brain structures such as the cerebral cortex, the micturition center governs voluntary emptying of the urinary bladder (urination). From these few examples, one can see how important the brainstem is and why the effects of aging on it are of concern.

In August 2013 a forty-year-old male friend showed me MRIs of his cervical vertebral column and spinal cord and described neck pain he had been experiencing in the previous several weeks. He also mentioned having recently strained his shoulders and neck when he was moving heavy furniture for another friend and doing military presses with too much weight. Based on the MRIs and a consultation, an orthopedist had told my friend that he had bone spurs on the vertebrae at C3 and C4. One could clearly see in the MRIs that these were enlarged and were probably compressing both motor and sensory nerves in the region. I told my friend how important C3, C4, and adjacent areas are for communication between the regulatory centers of the brainstem and the spinal cord, in particular as these influence respiration. Cell bodies of the phrenic nerve (the main respiratory nerve that controls the diaphragm) make connections in this region with motor nerves that descend from the respiratory control centers in the brainstem. The orthopedist had told my friend that his neck pain and inflammation would only get worse with time and that there was nothing that the doctor could do. I suggested that my friend avoid shoulder or neck workouts, give the tissue time to heal, and contact a sports medicine specialist who might be able to treat the swelling and pain with anti-inflammatory medications. In the past I had experienced such relief from treatments by my physician, who understands sports medicine. My friend agreed with my suggestion, sought help from a sports medicine specialist, and some months later was feeling much improved.

The Aging Brainstem and Hearing

According to *Dorland's Illustrated Medical Dictionary*, presbycusis (pres-bē-cūsis) is a progressive, bilaterally symmetrical loss of hearing that occurs with age. Currently, there is no effective medication to prevent or treat presbycusis. Although cochlear implants can effectively replace the mechanical and sensory functions of lost hair cells by providing direct electrical stimulation to spiral ganglion neurons, this technique will be successful only when sufficient numbers of these hearing-related neurons remain. Thus, with the continuous increase of the elderly population around the world, there is an urgent need to understand the causes of the loss of spiral ganglion neurons with age.

Age-related loss of spiral ganglion neurons is consistently observed in humans and animals. In humans, the age-related loss of these neurons, while the organ of Corti is relatively unaffected, is classified as neural presbycusis. Not all loss of spiral ganglion neurons is debilitating, nor do all cases of it merit a label of neural presbycusis. Most of us are born with a surplus of spiral ganglion neurons—maybe ten times the number needed to detect sounds, and perhaps twice the number needed to make fine distinctions between multiple frequencies. A definitive label of neural presbycusis requires an accelerated loss of spiral ganglion neurons that progressively impairs one's perception of sound at a rate that exceeds the physiological age of the individual. The early manifestations of this can include decreased speech intelligibility, especially in noisy environments, poor signal-to-noise ratios, and impaired resolution of frequency. The latter problem can contribute to an individual's impaired ability to identify the source of natural sounds and probably alters the quality of music they hear. The fact that not everyone exhibits neural presbycusis suggests that both genetic and environmental factors contribute to this condition. Thus, the survival of spiral ganglion neurons during aging is largely the result of genetic and environmental interactions. These complex interactions can be manifested at the systemic, cellular, and molecular levels.

Loss of hearing is the most common sensory deficit in the elderly and is becoming a serious social and health problem internationally. Especially in the elderly, loss of hearing can impair the exchange of information and significantly affect everyday life, causing loneliness, isolation, dependence, and frustration, as well as communication problems (for example, hearing "she already took her medication" instead of "Shanese booked this summer's vacation"). Loss of hearing (as opposed to injury or acute or chronic disease) is the most common cause of adult hearing deficiency and is considered the most prevalent sensory impairment in the elderly (seventy-five years and older). In the United States loss of hearing affects 40 percent of the population seventy-five years of age and older. Recent estimates suggest that by 2030 35 to 40 million senior citizens in the United States could have significant hearing loss.

Fewer than 40 percent of adults with impaired hearing perceive that they have an excellent overall quality of life or very good physical health. This compares to nearly 70 percent of those without hearing loss. Almost one-third of people with impaired hearing report being in fair or poor health, compared to only 9 percent of people with no loss of hearing. Thus, the elderly with loss of hearing are less satisfied with their life than people without impaired hearing. As a result of failing communication abilities, people with loss of hearing perceive their social skills as poor, and they often experience reduced self-esteem. Loss of hearing in particular is reported to be a source of loneliness, isolation, decline in social activities, and dissatisfaction with family life.

Loss of hearing with age is not experienced exclusively by humans. The other species that also suffer from the malady are particularly useful in researching the topic. Through research with such animals, we have learned that the auditory pons is an important location for the development and maintenance of hearing. Structures in the pons—including the cochlear nucleus and calyx of Held (a large nerve terminal that is located in the auditory brainstem and is involved in sound localization)—and their regulation of hearing have been under intense investigation in recent decades. Globular bushy cells at the bottom of the cochlear nucleus project upward to the medial nucleus, where their large axons terminate on cell bodies of the latter neurons, forming the calyx of Held. Current research is aimed at better understanding how electrical and signaling activity in the presynaptic terminal affects the release of neurotransmitters in the brain. The calyx of Held allows investigators to make pre- and postsynaptic recordings of nerve activity. This aids them in studying many presynaptic activities, including electrical currents and their effects on synaptic transmission.

A major limitation for experiments on mice using the calyx of Held is that electrical recordings are typically limited to days six to fourteen after birth, which might not be indicative of adult or aging function. One difficulty in using older mice to make these recordings is simply visualizing the calyx of Held. To solve this problem, some investigators use precision microtomes (scientific cutting instruments) to make 100-micrometer (one tenth of a millimeter) thin slices of the extracted pons rather than the typical 170-micrometer slices used in other lines of neuroscience experimentation. In addition, due to the decreased surface area in the calyx of Held of older animals, it is still technically challenging to obtain presynaptic recordings. To bypass this limitation, investigators attempt to record from the region where the neurons expand to form the calyx. Lines of research like these are important because establishing techniques for recording from adult animal brains leads to a better understanding of presynaptic function in physiological and pathological conditions in older animals and humans. Although recordings from aging animals are difficult to make, they allow investigators to study changes in presynaptic activity that occur over time.

Another technique for studying loss of hearing in aging animals is to count the numbers of hearing-related cells. Such cell counts have shown substantial decreases in the number of neurons in the auditory pons of aging rats. This effect of aging seems to be specific to selected nuclei because the numbers of cells and nuclei in adjacent areas remain unchanged in rodents from three to thirty months of age. This might be explained on the basis that neurons of some nuclei are more susceptible to death than neurons in other nuclei because they have fewer excitatory inputs. Also, the continuing expression of specific proteins in selected neurons decreases in some strains of mice with age-related loss of hearing. Degeneration of axons and other lesions become prominent in the same hearing-related nuclei of old gerbils. All these changes might contribute to the diminution of sound in aging animals and could be relevant to the loss of hearing in humans.

Elderly people who have impaired hearing often feel left out in group settings and conversations. Consider the last wedding reception you attended. By the time the meal is served, the wedding ceremony is already two to three hours in the past. In the interim the open or cash bar has been packed with visitors, mostly in their twenties to forties. After a few hours of drinking, they can be partially or fully intoxicated, loud, and obnoxious. Add to their commotion the constant noise of prerecorded music or a band, as well as conversation at and between tables. The aging who are hearing impaired are often ignored and feel isolated. They are easily identified by their apparent age and the fact that they are usually sitting alone, somber and withdrawn.

In the years between 2003 and 2010, my wife and I made frequent trips to the Intermountain West to visit our aging parents and other family members. These were times for our extended families to gather in their homes or nearby public parks for picnics, grilling food, and visiting. Such gatherings always included a large handful of twenty- to sixty-year-old adults (our parents' children) and their young and adolescent children and grandchildren. We younger adults were so often preoccupied visiting with each other that we unintentionally ignored both our children and our parents. As our fathers aged, my wife and I both noticed them withdraw from these family gatherings and noisy conversations. My wife asked her father about his lack of participation. He remarked that because of the continuous background noise he could not hear the conversations, didn't know what was being discussed, and felt excluded. I regret my own contribution to his withdrawal, and the lack of sensitivity and consideration so often displayed by clamoring, attention-seeking younger adults.

One of the mechanisms by which aging impairs hearing is through the insulin or insulin-like growth factor pathway and the generation of calories. We live in a time of overeating and in a nation of ubiquitous food establishments. There are restaurants on almost every corner, fast food at our fingertips, and seemingly insatiable appetites for all kinds of things to eat. Overeating causes elevations in the production of insulin and insulin-like growth factors. These lead to increased oxidation of carbohydrates, fats, and proteins and to elevated production of the damaging oxidants discussed in chapter 1. The evidence that overeating impairs hearing and accelerates the aging process is that undereating does the opposite in both animals and humans. Therefore, one effective way to regulate the insulin and insulin-like growth factor pathways is through restricting calories, which has been shown in multiple species to extend longevity.

Self-disciplined restrictions in food consumption result in significant alterations in circulating concentrations of insulin-like growth factor 1. Such discipline helps regulate the neuroendocrine axis during aging. Restricting the intake of calories enhances plasticity of the brain (growth of new cells) and also delays the age-related loss of neurons in the enteric nervous system. Restricting the intake of calories modulates mitochondrial function in nerve tissue, leading to decreased production and release of reactive oxygen species. Reducing consumption of food also increases tissue levels of neuroprotective factors and molecular chaperones, as well as decreasing the activity of pro-apoptotic and inflammatory chemicals. In an extensive study on cochlear aging in multiple strains of mice, restricting food intake was found to ameliorate age-related loss of spiral ganglion neurons. These and related studies suggest that food restriction can delay the onset of loss of hearing with age. More work is needed to determine if there is a gender component to these findings and how they might vary among various cultures and ethnic groups.

When I wrote this chapter, my mother was in her mid-eighties and had been suffering for several years from loss of vision and hearing. I had been diagnosed with right-sided vocal cord paralysis. My mother lives in Utah and I live in New Jersey. We don't see each other often enough. Our main channels of communication have been the phone and handwritten letters. However, as my voice weakens and her hearing declines, telephone communication has become increasingly difficult for us. Now in our phone calls, one of her most frequent comments is "Huh?" My usual response is to repeat what I had just said, only louder. A ten- or fifteen-minute phone call of this sort reduces my vocal volume and endurance for the next several days. I have come to question the success of our conversations.

The Aging Pons and Urination

Beyond vision and hearing, one of the physiological tasks we engage in regularly is urinating. This is true for both men and women, and the number of daily trips to the bathroom increases with age in many of us. I will have more to say about this in chapter 6. Still, age-related enlargement of the prostate gland in men and overactivity of the bladder in women can have some elderly people on edge during most of their waking hours. This is especially true when the periods between bathroom visits can be as long as several hours (for example, on cruise ships with malfunctioning restrooms, on crowded coast-to-coast and international flights, in lengthy meetings or worship services, and at sporting events). Under these conditions, careful planning is needed more as we age than when we were younger. Knowing where the nearest bathroom is can almost be lifesaving.

Difficulties of the lower urinary tract occur in 15–60 percent of men over age forty in the United States and Europe, and the prevalence of such symptoms rises markedly with age. In the Boston Area Community Health Study, the prevalence of these problems increased from 8 percent of men in their thirties to 35 percent of men in their sixties. Similarly, in one international study the prevalence increased 10 percent per decade, from ages forty to seventy-nine years. Nocturnal urination (nocturia) is such a commonplace occurrence in the lives of many older adults that it is frequently overlooked as a potential cause of sleep disturbance and fall-induced injury. When people were asked about it, 53 percent listed nocturia as a cause of disrupted sleep every night or almost every night. This was more than four times greater than the 12 percent who listed pain, the next most frequently cited cause of poor sleep. Every nocturnal trip to the bathroom represents a potentially serious fall. Regardless of the time of day, urge incontinence has been associated with falling, and evidence shows that nocturia itself is a risk factor for falling. Over an interval of five years, individuals who void two times a night are at twice the risk of falling as those who do not get up at all, and the risk is even higher with three or more bathroom visits per night. In fact, three or more urinations per night increase the risk for fractures of the hip by 80 percent.

In older women overactive bladder is an especially common and troublesome problem. Typically it is associated with overactivity of the detrusor (layers of visceral smooth muscle that line the body of the urinary bladder), but the origins of that overactivity are frequently unknown. Urgency—an abnormal sensation in the bladder—signifies impending or actual loss of control and carries the emotional fear of leaking urine.

Imagine yourself in the following situation. You are attending an international conference. You have your breakfast between 7:00 and 8:00 A.M. and then walk several blocks to the convention center to attend a 9 A.M. keynote address. The room is in an unfamiliar part of the center, filled to capacity, and the speaker is midway through her talk about 9:15 A.M. You have already felt the first urges to urinate but don't want to miss anything. Unexpectedly, a fire alarm sounds. The building is evacuated, and you have to stand outside in the cold. Because you are standing (as opposed to sitting) the urgency to urinate intensifies. By the time the building's safety has been established and you are readmitted, it is 10:00 A.M. and now your need to find a bathroom is more than urgent. There isn't one in sight, and you frantically hurry through the crowded halls, trying not to be too conspicuous. Still you see no bathroom signs. It is most likely that by this time you have already begun to leak, drizzle, or otherwise wet yourself. If you are wearing absorbable panties and the volume of urine is low, you could be okay. In any case, you will feel

uncomfortable and will have to return to the hotel for a change of
clothing.

Control of the bladder is exercised by the central nervous system via a
long-loop spinal cord reflex that includes the pons of the brainstem, the
midbrain, and higher cerebral components. This network is similar to that
involved in the brain-gut interaction. Among the best understood and
most thoroughly investigated of these brain regions are: the periaqueduc-
tal gray matter, believed to receive the bladder's afferent signals via the
spinal cord; the insula, especially on the right side—activation of which is
linked to subjective visceral sensations (differing states of feeling); and
the dorsal anterior cingulate cortex, which is responsible for emotional
responses, motivational behaviors, and concurrent efferent autonomic
control. In these regions, especially in the insula, responses to filling of
the bladder during the storage of urine become stronger with increasing
volume and stretch. In addition, the prefrontal cortex is involved in urination. The medial part in particular is believed to be responsible for decisions such as whether to void or not, based on the social situation. Finally,
if voluntary voiding occurs, there is activation of the anterior cingulate
cortex and of the micturition control center (in the pons) that results in
coordinated relaxation of the urethral sphincters and contraction of the
detrusor muscle, and thus urination. Normal sensations associated with
filling of the bladder and desire to void include sensory feedback from the
distended bladder to the spinal cord and the higher brain locations just
mentioned. All of these are influenced by aging.

Aging-related changes in the normal brain-bladder control system,
and differences by age in urge incontinence in women ages twenty-six to
eighty-five years have been the focus of several clinical investigations.
Outcomes that these studies have measured include age-related brain
responses to artificial filling of the bladder (using functional MRI to map
brain structures that are involved), volume of the bladder, urge incontinence (manually compressing the abdomen over the distended bladder),
and overactivity of the detrusor muscle. Responses and their dependence
on age have been determined with small and large volumes in the bladder
and in the whole brain and in selected cerebral regions of interest
including the right insula and anterior cingulate (regions of the cerebrum
that are above and anterior to the brainstem). In control subjects, increasing

the volume of fluid in the bladder and noting corresponding sensations of fullness were accompanied by increasing responses in the insula detected by the MRI. With increasing age the detected responses became weaker. In younger women, the anterior cingulate responded with unusual strength at large volumes and sensations in the bladder. In elderly women, the response was strong at small volumes but reduced at large volumes. Activation of the micturition center in the pons did not differ between young and older women if detrusor overactivity was present.

In mice two to twenty-six months of age (young to old), maximum pressure inside the bladder, estimated strength of contraction of detrusor muscle, the time interval during which the detrusor is contracting, as well as indices of detrusor power and work did not decrease with age, suggesting that the mechanics of the bladder wall are sustained throughout the life cycle in this species. However, the intervals between urinations (the inter-urination interval), volumes of urine eliminated, and urine flow rates at each voiding decreased with age. Additionally, calculations of the tension that developed in the wall of the bladder during filling suggested the loss of sensitivity to changes in volume in the aging bladder. Such investigations conclude that aging is associated with an impaired ability to respond to the challenge of continuous filling of the bladder.

The Aging Autonomic Nervous System: Sympathetic Changes

In 1920 Walter B. Cannon, a renowned American physiologist who was chairman of the Department of Physiology at Harvard Medical School, said the autonomic nervous system is essential for maintaining physiological balance of the organism—a process he named "homeostasis." Today we know that the autonomic nervous system is an important neuroregulator of cardiovascular, endocrine, gastrointestinal, metabolic, respiratory, and many other functions in humans and other mammals. The rates of cardiovascular disease morbidity and mortality increase markedly with advancing age, and aging is a physiological process related to structural and functional changes in the cardiovascular and autonomic nervous systems that lead to coronary vascular disease, heart failure, hypertension, myocardial infarction, and stroke. Consequently, medical and scientific literature suggests that aging is a risk factor for cardiovascular disease. In addition, environmental factors and sedentary lifestyles can increase the effects of aging on the autonomic nervous system and to cardiovascular disease.

During the past several decades, changes in sympathetic function that occur with age in healthy adult humans have been investigated systematically using a combination of neurochemical, neurophysiological, and hemodynamic experimental approaches. The composite evidence from these investigations suggests that the tonic activity (the release of a neurotransmitter with time) of the sympathetic nervous system increases with age. Tonic activity is determined by the ability of these nerves to release neurotransmitters such as norepinephrine (noradrenalin), by an increase in peripheral vascular resistance to blood flow, and by elevations in heart rate in baseline, resting conditions. The elevations in sympathetic tone in the heart appear to be due, at least in part, to reductions in neuronal reuptake of norepinephrine and not necessarily to its increased release into the blood. Elevations in sympathetic nerve activity with age also appear to influence skeletal muscle and the gastrointestinal tract, but not the kidney.

In contrast to sympathetic nerve activity, tonic release of epinephrine (adrenalin) from the adrenal medulla is markedly reduced with age. This is not reflected in circulating plasma concentrations of epinephrine because of reduced plasma clearance (the removal of epinephrine from the plasma). And contrary to broadly held views, the acute stress-related responsiveness of the sympathetic nervous system and adrenal glands (the so-called sympathoadrenal discharge in fight-or-flight decisions) is not elevated with age in healthy adults. Indeed, the release of epinephrine in response to acute stress is noticeably attenuated in older men. The mechanisms underlying the age-related increments in activity of the sympathetic nervous system have not been definitively established, but some evidence points to an increase in drive from the subcortical central nervous system.

Because sympathetic nerve activity in skeletal muscle is representative of cerebral or subcortical activation of the sympathetic nervous system, the above results support the interpretation of a net increase in the release of norepinephrine as evidence for elevated central activation of the sympathetic nerves with human aging. The data also suggest that a primary target of the increased sympathetic activity is skeletal muscle in the limbs. If skeletal muscle is a primary target, then the vessels supplying blood flow to the extremities are also a target. This would help explain the elevations in blood pressure with age, particularly in sedentary adults. Related investigations on rigorously screened adults have demonstrated that: (1) sympathetic nerve activity in skeletal muscle increases with age even in healthy adults without established high blood pressure, suggesting a primary effect of physiological aging; (2) sympathetic nerve activity in skeletal muscle doubles between the ages of twenty-five and sixty-five in healthy adults; (3) the increase is observed in both men and women; and (4) the age-related increments in sympathetic nerve activity are not always observable using measurements of norepinephrine in antecubital venous plasma (that is, measuring concentrations of norepinephrine in the blood is not always consistent with the activity of sympathetic nerves).

Besides collecting blood samples and measuring concentrations of neurotransmitters in them, there is another method for estimating activity of the sympathetic nervous system: microneurography. This is a technique in which miniature devices, including electrodes like the needles used in acupuncture, are placed near major sympathetic nerve tracts that innervate skeletal muscle. Microneurographic images are then taken of the frequency and intensity of nerve activity in these tracts under baseline conditions and during experimental maneuvers. Age-induced hypertension is associated with images revealing increased sympathetic nerve activity.

A significant limitation of this imaging technique, however, is that it cannot be used on internal organs. To acquire additional insights about internal organs, investigators must perform alternative experiments. In one such study, researchers found that the rate of release of cardiac norepinephrine into coronary venous plasma in healthy older men was almost double the amount in healthy younger men. This appeared to represent both increased cardiac sympathetic nerve activity and a reduction in the reuptake of norepinephrine. Similar results were found in circulation in the liver and gut but not in renal plasma samples. Collectively, the evidence supports the view that aging in humans is associated with a net activation of the sympathetic nervous system.

The discharge of sympathetic nerves innervating the skin is reduced in aged compared with middle-aged and young human subjects. This reduction poses problems because blood flow to selected areas of the skin plays an important role in regulating body temperature. If these neurogenic thermoregulatory mechansims are impaired by age, then engaging in heat-producing activities might be more dangerous for older individuals. For example, doing heavy yard work on a hot, humid day in July or August might cause your body to generate and store heat more rapidly than it can get rid of it. This will lead to an elevation in body temperature and possibly to heat exhaustion or heat stroke. One sign that you are overdoing things is if you are losing a great deal of fluid through sweating.

In early July 2013, I was using my chain saw to remove large tree branches that were hanging over my shed. It was hot and humid, and I worked hard for about sixty minutes. I had weighed myself that morning before starting, and I did so again after completing the job and cooling down. I knew I had lost a lot of water because of my soaked T-shirt and the moisture in the towel I used to dry my forehead. After weighing myself the second time, I found that I had lost about six pounds (for a rate of 0.6 milliliters per kilogram each minute), despite drinking water a couple of times during those sixty minutes of hard work.

It has been thought for many years that aging humans display sympathetic hyperactivity to acute stress. However, recent research on young and older subjects indicates that their responses to acute stressors are similar. But because resting rates of discharge (the firing of nerve action potentials) are higher in older subjects, relative increments in discharge during acute stress are reduced. Other research suggests that aging attenuates sympathetic discharge to muscle when selected cardiovascular reflexes are activated. Similarly, stress-induced release of epinephrine from the adrenal medulla was reduced in older men when compared with younger men. These findings support the view that human aging is unlikely to cause heightened sympathoadrenal activation during acute stress.

The cold pressor test is an acute challenge to the sympathetic nervous system and has been used to diagnose cardiovascular disease. For example, it has been proposed as a way of identifying young adults who might be at increased risk of cardiovascular disease as they age. We have used this test in Systems Physiology Laboratory at Rutgers University to help teach students cardiovascular physiology. The test consists of having volunteer subjects immerse either a hand (or a foot) in water chilled to about 0–4° centigrade. If the subject is going to immerse a hand, we first attach a thermistor at the base of the thumb. This allows us to estimate skin temperature during immersion. We also attach a standard limb lead electrocardiogram (ECG) and a blood pressure cuff. Then we ask the subject to immerse the hand with the thermistor and leave it in place for three minutes. We collect data before, during, and after the hand is immersed. Only volunteers are used, and we try to obtain an equal number of young men and young women.

In the average subject, both blood pressure and heart rate increase modestly but significantly by the end of immersion. In about one-quarter to one-third of the volunteers we see exaggerated blood pressure responses. In these cases, both systolic and diastolic pressures rise to values that are three to four times those of the average subjects. The literature suggests that this might be indicative of a predisposition to cardiovascular disease later in life in such individuals. We do our best to minimize these subjects' fear and worry, but if/when they ask for advice, we encourage them to report the findings to their physician and to consider consulting a cardiologist.

Central neural mechanisms mediating age-associated changes in the rate of discharge of sympathetic nerves remain largely unknown. Some investigators have measured the turnover (rates of production and degradation) of norepinephrine in selected regions of the central nervous system under baseline conditions in young and aging men and have reported increased rates in the turnover of norepinephrine in older men. These increases in turnover were accompanied by increased appearance of norepinephrine in venous blood coming from the heart, liver, and mesentery (gut). More research is needed on age-related changes in baroreceptor sensitivity and the discharge of sympathetic nerves in skeletal muscle of humans. However, investigators have reported that older subjects demonstrate reduced sympathetic activation when blood pressure is reduced in the carotid sinus. Conversely, when sinus pressure was increased, elderly subjects displayed greater inhibition of sympathetic discharge to blood vessels in skeletal muscle.

The Aging Autonomic Nervous System:
Parasympathetic Changes

Aging is known to alter the neurohormonal mechanisms that control the cardiovascular system, and cardiovascular diseases are associated with autonomic changes that include a decrease in parasympathetic and/or an increase in sympathetic output. The sinoatrial node (or natural pacemaker of the heart) is a case in point. Pacemaker cells in the node set the cardiac rhythm. They have the quality of automaticity—that is, changing membrane electrical activity that is unique and innate to these cells. This means the pacemaker cells are able to depolarize and repolarize (discharge and recharge) independent of any external stimuli, including that from parasympathetic and sympathetic nerves. Autonomic nerves influence pacemaker activity but do not determine it.

Under normal conditions in healthy people, the vagus nerves (parasympathetic) play a major role in determining resting heart rate, especially in physically fit individuals. Impairment in the function of cardiac vagus nerves appears to be one of the major determinants of changes in the control of heart rate with age. For example, aging reduces the elevations in heart rate that are seen following the administration of atropine in humans and animals (drug-induced tachycardia). Atropine is a synthetic antagonist that blocks the ability of acetylcholine, the main neurotransmitter released by parasympathetic nerves such as the vagus, to bind to its corresponding receptor on cardiac pacemaker cells. In animal experiments, young rats showed a lower intrinsic heart rate after administration of atropine than did older rats. This suggests that there were more atropine-sensitive receptors to block in young rats and that the number of receptors had diminished in aging animals. Similar experiments in young and old people demonstrated smaller increments in the elderly in heart rate, cardiac output, systolic blood pressure, and early diastolic filling, suggesting deteriorating influences of the vagus nerves with age.

Respiratory sinus arrhythmia is a phrase used to describe the influence of the rhythmicity of breathing on the function of the cardiac pacemaker. Under normal conditions heart rate, blood flow, and blood pressure rise modestly during inspiration and decline during expiration.

This is because respiration affects the rate of venous blood flow returning to the heart (venous return). Venous return influences the filling of the atria with blood, and therefore the stretch applied to atrial walls. Such atrial filling affects important reflexes that participate in the central regulation of both circulation and respiration.

Attenuation of respiratory sinus arrhythmia with age suggests the loss of the parasympathetic nerves' influence on the sinoatrial node. Moreover, beneficial autonomic, cardiovascular, endocrine, and metabolic changes associated with frequent exercise demonstrate that regular physical activity is an important intervention that can minimize unwanted cardiac changes associated with aging. Thus, regular exercise in animals and humans results in adaptation of the autonomic nervous system that is most commonly observed as a significant reduction in resting heart rate. This is thought to be mediated by an increase in the rates of discharge of the vagus nerves that innervate the sinoatrial node.

How exactly is a reduction in one's resting heart rate related to beneficial health-related consequences? Each time the heart contracts, it performs physical work. In its simplest definition, work is the ability of a force to move a load over a distance. In the heart, load is the equivalent of stroke volume (mass of blood) ejected during each cardiac cycle. Stroke volume or load must be moved over a distance (for example, out of the ventricle and into the aorta) by a force (strength of ventricular contraction). This cardiac work, like all manual labor, requires the expenditure of energy during each cardiac cycle. The fewer times a heart contracts per unit of time—that is, the fewer cycles there are—the less work is done over time. This translates into reduced wear and tear on the heart and thus to cardiac preservation. The take-home message is that regular physical activity is good for the heart because it reduces resting heart rate and conserves energy.

The Aging Peripheral Nervous System

All skeletal muscles are innervated by somatic motor nerves. The numbers, size, and physiological functioning of motor nerves diminish with age. Therefore, age-related loss of motor nerves, muscle mass, and physical function greatly affects quality of life in the elderly. A motor unit consists of a single motor nerve and all the muscle fibers it innervates. The greater the strength or frequency of a stimulus applied to a motor nerve, the greater the number of muscle fibers activated. This is called muscle recruitment. Perhaps a stimulus strength of one millivolt to a nerve will be sufficient to recruit ten muscle fibers that can collectively move a load of ten pounds. But a stimulus strength of ten millivolts will recruit many more muscle fibers—perhaps one hundred—and therefore should move a much heavier load—say, a hundred pounds.

Loss of motor nerve activity with age can be thought of as functional denervation (as opposed to surgical or chemical denervation). Several hypotheses have been proposed to account for age-related loss of function of motor nerves, but accumulating evidence points to alterations at the neuromuscular junction as the main cause of aging-related muscle wasting and general weakness. The neuromuscular junction is a complex system composed of a presynaptic motor nerve, a synapse or synaptic cleft, and a motor endplate (the region of the postsynaptic muscle fiber that is innervated by the presynaptic motor neuron). It is not unreasonable to suspect that aging can affect any or all of these structures and the cellular or molecular events that occur at each. For example, on the presynaptic side of the junction, the motor neuron terminus contains vesicles that store and release neurotransmitters. Without the vesicles and neurotransmitters there could be no postsynaptic muscle response. Similarly, on the postsynaptic side of the junction, the muscle cell membrane (sarcolemma) contains protein receptors that recognize neurotransmitters and act as docking stations for them. Both of these systems, as well as multiple others, are subject to the effects of aging.

During the past few decades, aging-associated degeneration of the neuromuscular junction and its components has been well documented. With advancing age, presynaptic motor axons exhibit regions of abnormal thinning, distension, and sprouting, whereas the number of postsynaptic endplates decreases—as do their size, length, and density of post-synaptic folds. Postsynaptic folds and surface area are directly proportional. The greater the number of folds, the larger the surface area. Greater surface area means more receptor docking sites. Therefore, the greater the number of postsynaptic folds, the greater the potential number of neurotransmitter binding sites.

Although the precise mechanisms are unknown, recent evidence suggests that aging-related increments in cellular oxidative stress play a critical role in the degenerating neuromuscular junction, and thus in the progression of muscle wasting. For example, experimental deletion of the important antioxidant enzyme superoxide dismutase in young animals causes accelerated age-dependent muscle atrophy and degeneration of the neuromuscular junction. The change is similar to that seen in old animals of the same body type but with aging-related muscle degeneration. More specifically, reductions in the numbers of presynaptic vesicles, mitochondria, and surface area were reported in both soleus and extensor digitorum longus muscles from twenty-nine-month-old mice (aged mice) compared to those from mice only seven months old. Soleus and extensor digitorum longus muscles in the limbs that are involved in mobility (such as running and jumping). On the postsynaptic side of the junction, in older mice there is an increase in the number of folds and an increased number of vesicles beneath the cell membrane.

It has also been hypothesized that age-related changes in the neuro-muscular junction are associated with alterations in the transport of materials down the axons. For example, a decline in axonal transport during aging could affect the availability of growth factors as well as movement of subcellular organelles, such as mitochondria, that are crucial for the function and survival of motor neurons. In one experiment, axonal transport was compared in young, middle-aged, and old male rats by measuring the accumulation of cholinesterase at the neuromuscular junction in the injured sciatic nerve (a knot was tied in the nerve to impair its function). Accumulation of the enzyme was significantly reduced in older rats, suggesting that transport from cell bodies was attenuated by the injury.

Mammalian axons, their associated Schwann cells, and related cell types of the peripheral nervous system function in a special environment: the endoneurial microenvironment. Exchange of material between this physiological space and the interstitium (that is, general extracellular space) is restricted and regulated by a blood-nerve barrier known as the blood-nerve interface. The blood-nerve interface consists of the vascular endothelium of blood vessels (inside the cellular lining) and a multilayered nerve sheath surrounding axons and Schwann cells called the perineurium. The relative impermeability of this barrier to blood-borne

materials protects the endoneurial microenvironment from harmful constituents of plasma and from rapid fluctuations in concentrations of
plasma solutes, which could adversely affect the microenvironment and its
physiological properties. Moreover, the absence of lymphatic drainage of
the endoneurial space emphasizes the protective nature of the blood-
nerve interface because, apart from the cerebrum and central nervous system, this is one of the few physiological spaces known to lack lymphatic
vessels.

The sympathetic nerve activity of skeletal muscle is not only affected
by age, but it also differs between men and women. Both the frequency and
incidence of bursts of electrical activity in these nerves increases with age.
Men, both young and older, have greater sympathetic nerve activity in
skeletal muscle than women of the corresponding ages. This means,
among other things, that the resistance to blood flow in the vasculature of
such muscles is greater in men than in women, which could help explain
why blood pressure in men is usually higher than in women.

Nerve membranes seem to be comparably permeable in the old and
the young. Therefore, it is of interest to learn how developing nerves in
young people avoid the aging-and disease-related problems observed in
nerves of older adults. In older adults, movement of proteins out of
the blood leads to edema and inflammation. This results mainly from
albumin-induced elevation of oncotic or protein osmotic pressure in the
endoneurial interstitial space. Albumin and other proteins such as the
immunoglobulins attract ions and water, creating oncotic pressure. Water
drawn oncotically into the endoneurial interstitium from the vascular
compartment leads to increased endoneurial water content and, together
with low perineurial compliance, causes an elevation in hydrostatic
pressure in this space.

The increased hydrostatic pressure and accompanying extravascular
and extraneuronal compression occludes blood vessels and compresses
nerves that supply the endoneurial microcirculation and its environs. In
contrast, a highly permeable blood-nerve interface during neonatal development does not lead to edema and elevated hydrostatic pressure because
the perineurium is more permeable, which prevents the endoneurial
accumulation of fluids and osmols (electrolytes and ions attached to proteins that give the proteins their water-drawing potential). In addition,

greater compliance (the ability of a tissue to stretch without a corresponding increase in tension or pressure) of the endoneurium in young people
minimizes elevations in hydrostatic pressure in this compartment. Thus,
the need for greater blood-nerve exchange of material to support growth,
among other things, likely promotes a more permeable endoneurial
microvasculature in young, developing nerves.

At the other end of the growth spectrum, the integrity and microenvironment of the blood-nerve interface have been studied in animals. Permeability to sugars in the sciatic nerve and vascular space and water
content of the tibial nerve were assessed in rats three to thirty months of
age, with no age-dependent differences observed. This suggests that once
established in early adulthood, the integrity of the blood-nerve interface
is not altered, even in aged rats. Conversely, aging is associated with
increased hydrostatic pressure in the epineurium, which has been shown
to have two developmental plateaus: the first from about one to four
months of age and the second from six months onward. The first increase
is associated with appearance of the blood-nerve interface in young adults,
while the second seems to be associated with the age-dependent reductions in compliance of the perineurium. Thickening of the basement
membranes of perineurial cells has been observed in patients with diabetes and in the aging. This might be a structural correlate of the reduced
compliance of perineurial sheaths.

Aging and Eyesight

The critical role of the eyes in good health has become increasingly
evident. Sunlight, eyesight, and good health are compatible partners.
I spent the months of January, February, and March 1967 in Fort Lewis,
Washington, during basic training in the US Army. This was the rainy
season, and members of my platoon were frequently hospitalized for
weather-related illnesses because we were almost always wet. At one point,
I counted thirty-two consecutive days during which I did not see the sun.
It was a depressing experience for this enlisted man, because it was my
first exposure to such limited sunlight.

Exposure to natural sunlight (environmental illumination) is
inversely correlated to conditions such as insomnia and depression, both

of which increase with age. Chronic insomnia and depression are closely associated. Disturbances in sleep that are chronic affect 40–70 percent of the elderly. In one recent study, only 12 percent of 9,000 subjects ages sixty-five and older said they had no complaints about loss of sleep. Correspondingly, about 30 percent of older adults have depression. Depression, like insomnia, frequently goes undiagnosed in this age group. Moreover, insomnia and depression are significant risk factors for cancer, cardiovascular disease, cognitive deficiencies, dementia, diabetes, and premature mortality.

Both the production and release of melatonin increase in natural light, and melatonin appears to be an anti-aging hormone. Its daily concentrations in the circulating plasma are cyclic. The nocturnal concentrations of the hormone are reduced with aging in some but not all people, probably because of differences in their exposure to environmental sunlight. Reduced concentrations of circulating melatonin are also associated with higher risks of cancer and other diseases. Bright light (that is, greater than 2,500 lux, which is explained below)—particularly from blue sources such as outdoor daylight—can reduce or eliminate insomnia and depression. It can increase alertness, brain serotonin levels, and cognitive function and can improve mood. Moreover, regular exposure to sunlight can stabilize the extremes in peaks and valleys of hormones, including nocturnal concentrations of melatonin that might have been previously undetectable (prior to increased exposure to natural light).

It is a rare sunny day when I don't spend at least thirty to sixty minutes in the sun. On such days I walk to work, ride a bicycle during lunch, or simply watch people from a bench directly exposed to sunlight in one of my favorite spots on campus. I have loved the sunshine all my life, and I don't ever recall being depressed.

Lux is the International System unit of illuminance that measures luminous flux per unit area. It is equal to one lumen per square meter. In photometry, the lux is used as a measure of the intensity, as perceived by the human eye, of light that hits or passes through a surface. One can think of luminous flux (measured in lumens) as a measure of the total amount of visible light present, and the illuminance as a measure of the intensity of illumination on a surface. A given amount of light will illuminate a surface more dimly if it is spread over a larger area, so illuminance is inversely proportional to area. A flux of 1,000 lumens concentrated onto an area of one square meter lights up the area with an illuminance of 1,000 lux. However, the same 1,000 lumens spread out over ten square meters produces a dimmer illuminance of only 100 lux. Thus, lighting a larger area to the same level of lux requires a greater number of lumens.

Young adults in industrialized countries typically receive only 20–120 minutes of exposure to daily light exceeding 1,000 lux. This is not intentional exposure to healthy sunlight. It represents time spent darting between the house and car, the bus or train terminal and the office, the office and the gym, and other sun-evading acts of life. Few such people get their daily exposures to sunlight by purposely planning it. Worse, the exposure of older adults to bright light (including sunlight) averages less than half that of young adults. Even more discouraging is the fact that institutionalized older people receive less than ten minutes of exposure to bright light exceeding 1,000 lux per day, with median light intensities as low as 50 lux. The declining exposure to sunlight of many older adults, combined with their reduced retinal capacity to absorb light due to pupillary miosis and yellowing of the crystalline lens, places them at increased risk for deficiencies in retinal photoreception. This could contribute to age-related cognitive decline, depression, and insomnia.

While I was researching parts of this book in 2011–13, I routinely walked from the College Avenue Campus to the Busch Campus at Rutgers University. The distance is two and a half miles each way. My office is on the Busch Campus, so this forced me at the end of the day to walk back to College Avenue to retrieve my parked car. Whenever possible, I timed my walks in both directions to correspond with the rising and setting of the sun. On clear, dark mornings and evenings this purposeful effort often allowed me to follow the rhythms of the waxing or waning moon and to view planets and stars.

On Wednesday, November 28, 2012, I had an unusual experience. I remember the date because it was when a dear friend died. Walking to my office I watched a full moon set in the west just about fifteen to twenty minutes before the sun rose in the east. Later that evening, while driving home, I saw the setting sun a couple hours before the reappearance of the full moon in the southeast. Thus, in less than fourteen hours I witnessed these four celestial events and was filled with awe, inspiration, and a deep sense of gratitude for life and all it has offered me.

My feelings as I watch a sunrise or a waxing or waning moon are indescribable, and the earliest memories of this profound appreciation for natural light extend back to my youth. I had a summer job in the Teton National Forest, in Jackson Hole, Wyoming. It lasted from early June to mid-August after my sophomore and junior years in high school. We would camp in the east foothills, directly across the valley from the Grand Tetons and the Snake River. Our bosses woke us each morning between 5:00 and 5:30 A.M. By the time we got dressed, had breakfast, and were setting out for the day's work, the sun was rising in the east but still out of view. The sunlight colored those snow-capped peaks various shades of pink, salmon, and yellow. Late in the evenings, the sunsets seemed to deposit a layer of molten gold on those jagged crags. It comes as no surprise to me to learn of the importance of sunlight as we age. In fact, I find it impossible to believe that such effects are limited to the physical body alone.

The Aging Enteric Nervous System

The gastrointestinal tract is innervated by intrinsic enteric nerves and by sympathetic and parasympathetic motor and visceral sensory nerves, all of which are compromised by age. Age-related loss of neurons occurs in both the myenteric plexus and submucosal or Auerbach's plexus of the intestines (both of which are part of the gut's nervous system). The myenteric plexus is a network of nerves that lies between two layers—the circular and longitudinal—of visceral smooth muscle. Both layers of muscle are subject to the influences of myenteric nerves and are involved in the mechanical movements of the gut wall. When the circular layer of smooth muscle contracts, the luminal diameter decreases. Contraction of the longitudinal layer shortens the segment of contracting gut. Both types of contraction aid in the processes of absorbing, digesting, mixing, and moving the contents of our meals. They also assist with gastrointestinal secretions.

Loss of neurons in both plexuses begins in adulthood, increases over the rest of the life span, and is most marked in cholinergic neurons. Cholinergic neurons are those that release acetylcholine as their primary neurotransmitter. In the autonomic nervous system, this includes both parasympathetic and sympathetic preganglionic axons, as well as postganglionic axons in the parasympathetic nerves. In the somatic or peripheral nervous system wherever efferent motor neurons meet their intended effector (for example, a smooth muscle cell in the gut), they release acetylcholine as the primary neurotransmitter.

Age-related neurodegeneration in the enteric nervous system might be key to functional changes observed in the gut with advancing age. One study found a 37 percent loss of enteric neurons in the colons of people older than age sixty-five, compared to those of younger people. In another study, researchers examined the number of nerve cells present in the myenteric plexus, as well as the numbers of collagen and elastic fibers of the human colon, in two groups of participants: those ages twenty to thirty-five and those over sixty-five. The total number of neurons decreased and both collagen and elastin increased in the older participants. Such findings suggest that neurodegeneration contributes to the disturbed colonic motility seen in the aging population. Parallel losses of enteric glia also occur with age. The extent of losses varies in a mouth-to-anus direction, with the segments of the gastrointestinal tract closest to the anus being most seriously affected. Additionally, with aging both axonal swellings and dilated varicosities progressively accumulate in the sympathetic and parasympathetic motor nerves and in the dorsal roots of the enteric nervous system. Such changes affect the conduction of action potentials and transmission of neurotransmitters at synaptic junctions. These findings are consistent with the increased incidence of colon-related disorders in the elderly, including constipation.

In contrast to the effects of aging on gastrointestinal motor nerves, the aging of sensory nerves in the gastrointestinal tract has not received much attention from investigators. A survey of the history of this question illustrates the point. Nearly thirty-five years ago, a full fifty years after the earliest descriptions of visceral sensory nerves (afferents), investigators noted that almost nothing was known about structural changes in visceral sensory nerves related to aging, and that motor networks in the autonomic nervous system had received much more attention. Little has changed since that time, and this oversight cannot be rationalized on the basis that functional disturbances such as acid reflux, constipation, diarrhea, and irritable bowel syndrome are manifested on the motor side of the gut reflex arc.

Changes in the function of motor nerves are as easily produced by upstream disturbances or losses of the sensory limb of a reflex loop as they are by direct compromise of motor neurons. Furthermore, motor dysfunctions, whatever their root causes, are more likely to remain uncompensated for or uncorrected if the afferent nerves monitoring them are impaired. The sparse observations on structural changes include the facts that, with age, cell bodies in the gastrointestinal sensory nerves that emerge from both the nodose and dorsal root ganglia lose Nissl bodies (an important component of healthy sensory nerves in the gastrointestinal tract) and that they accumulate lipofucsin, inclusions, aggregates, and tangles (all markers of aphysiological sensory nerves). These effects are associated with corresponding impairments in the structural integrity of their target organs, suggesting that local changes in the nerve's growth environment might give rise to the aging innervation of the gut.

The protein alpha-synuclein is expressed in local enteric neurons and in all vagal preganglionic motor nerves to the gut. Aggregations or misfolded masses of alpha-synuclein occur in many of the age-related neuropathies in the intrinsic and extrinsic motor neurons of the gut, but they are not seen in vagal sensory nerves. However, these sensory nerves probably release other proteins that are susceptible to age-related misfolding and aggregations. In any case, it appears that aging of vagal afferent nerves in the gastrointestinal tract involves mechanisms that are different from those affecting motor nerves. This is particularly relevant to aging-related diseases such as Parkinson's disease, in which sensory components of the nervous system remain intact while visceral motor systems progressively degenerate.

Constipation is a gastrointestinal problem that affects people of all ages. However, it can be particularly problematic in infants, children, and the aging and is often a concern to their caretakers and physicians. In older people the sudden onset of constipation can occur with acute illness or unexplained changes in their diets. In contrast, chronic constipation usually has an insidious onset period of months or years, often dating to childhood. Symptoms can range from a mild, acute event that is remedied with a shift in fluid intake and diet to chronic conditions that require daily interventions with mixed results. Older people might unwittingly believe that constipation is a natural part of aging, and it can be—depending on one's diet, behavior, and personality. However, most clinicians agree that constipation is not a disease, but rather is a general condition of difficulty in moving the bowels.

Notwithstanding, both the clinical and the scientific literature have shown that patients and clinicians use different definitions for constipation. Clinicians consider the frequency of bowel movements, weight of stools, colonic transit time, total gut transit time, and anorectal manometry as measures for constipation. A commonly held belief among clinicians is that constipation is more often imagined than real. This seems to stem from the fact that the great majority of those complaining of constipation have a bowel movement more frequently than three times per week. The normal frequency of moving one's bowels has a wide range of variability because our lives have a wide range of variability. Some clinicians consider the usual range for moving one's bowels to be from one to three times per day to three times per week. Less than three times per week might be considered normal if it does not represent a change from baseline and moving one's bowels is not uncomfortable or painful.

Still, the frequency and difficulty of moving one's bowels depends importantly on diet and other behavior. For example, those who move their bowels more than once a day are more likely to be overeating than those who move their bowels every other day. At the opposite extreme, individuals who are unwisely restricting their consumption of food (for example, those with eating disorders such as anorexia nervosa) might move their bowels once every few weeks. This is probably as unhealthy as having frequent stools due to overeating. Additionally, people who consume diets that are high in fats and simple sugars are more likely to be constipated than those who have diets rich in complex carbohydrates such as soluble and insoluble fiber (that is, grains and vegetables). This applies to children whose parents allow them to overindulge in artificially sweetened beverages and fatty snack products and to avoid fruits, grains, and vegetables. And it is equally true of the aged, whether or not they are institutionalized.

Moreover, there are routine events in our lives that can lead to sudden and marked changes in the neuroregulation of bowel function. Consider, for example, the last time you took a commercial or international flight that lasted more than about four hours. Regardless of the periodicity of your bowel movements before the flight, you may have noticed a change after the flight. Similarly, try keeping records of your regularity before and after long road trips (that is, those taking two to four days of 400–600 miles per day). These events and their unstudied or unknown effects on your psychosomatic well-being, including enteric nerves and gut function, can affect the timing and consistency of your bowel movements for days to weeks after the travel.

Motility of the colon and transit time in the gut are similar in healthy older adults and healthy young adults. In contrast, elderly people with chronic illness who report constipation have a prolonged total gut transit time of four to nine days compared with the average of less than three days. Movement of stool through the descending and sigmoid segments of the colon is especially slow in these people. The least mobile elderly people who live in nursing homes and other care facilities have transit times of up to three weeks. When estimating gut transit times in the aging US population, one must also consider the increasing epidemic of obesity and overweight. Reason tells us that those who chronically overeat will move their bowels more frequently than those who undereat. Common sense also tells us that the latter move their bowels less frequently because of reduced contents. Restricting the intake of calories also enhances plasticity of the brain and delays age-related neuronal loss in the enteric nervous system. For more on the aging gastrointestinal system, see chapter 7.

Delaying the Effects of Aging on the Nervous System

For most of us the process of aging is inevitable. Happily, however, it is possible to delay its effects and reduce their severity. For example, higher education and a lifetime of learning delay both the onset and the rapidity of aging's effects on intelligence, learning, and memory. So it is prudent to stay intellectually engaged by experimenting, learning, reading, studying, and writing. To this end an ongoing study funded by the National Institute of Aging is following a group of 678 Roman Catholic nuns. Among other things, investigators have recorded the effects of aging on postmortem brain weight, size, and other characteristics. Other study materials include autobiographical essays written (shortly after joining the sisterhood) to describe the nuns' ideas about their positions and responsibilities.

Thus far the study's findings suggest that the number of ideas written about in those essays, coupled with the use of complex propositions, is significantly correlated with lower risks for developing Alzheimer's disease in old age. And lower numbers of ideas accompanied lower brain weights, greater atrophy of brain tissue, and more neurofibrillary tangles (all characteristics of Alzheimer's) in postmortem examinations. It seems that the earlier and more frequently one begins expressing ideas in writing, the less likely one is to develop neurodegenerative diseases.

Living a physically active life is a good way to delay or protect against aging of the nervous system. The variability of heart rate responses to various activities is a case in point, at least as far as the aging autonomic nervous system is concerned. The greater the variability in heart rate the less likely an aging person is to die from cardiovascular diseases such as myocardial infarction and sudden cardiac death. Also, lower heart rates under baseline conditions are healthier for us as we age than elevated heart rates. Engaging in any physical activity regularly tends to lower baseline resting heart rate. Becoming and staying physically active can be done by exercising regularly alone or with friends, either indoors or outside, and with or without an expensive gym membership.

In summary, it has been said that the most educated university professors (those with earned PhDs) are among the least likely to suffer dementia. In research-intense environments like Rutgers University, the responsibilities of such professors frequently center on writing for peer-reviewed publications. To fund their research, faculty members write grant proposals. Grant proposals require the successful expression of specific aims and hypotheses. Those who write the most frequently are among the most likely to get funded. The converse is equally true. When such investigators complete a funded research project, they write one or more manuscripts for peers and others to read. This requires the written expression of ideas and a convincing defense of one's conclusions.

The most prolific writers, during a career of forty to fifty years, publish more than 500 peer-reviewed articles. In addition, they write several hundred abstracts, book chapters, and related documents. When not occupied in these activities, faculty members are writing or rewriting lectures, laboratory experiment results, and bureaucratic documents to meet local, state, and federal mandates for research and teaching (for example, documents for institutional review boards, institutional animal care and use committees, radiation and environmental health and safety offices, and offices of research and sponsored programs). In other words, professors at institutions such as the members of the Association of American Universities are first and foremost writers. They are also readers, speakers, thinkers, teachers, and doers.

One of my favorite writers was Arthur C. Guyton, a cardiovascular physiologist. By the time his forty-plus-year research and teaching career ended (in an automobile accident that took his and his wife's lives) he had written more than 600 peer-reviewed scientific manuscripts, published more than forty textbooks on physiology, and produced an untold number of related articles. He and his wife also had ten children, most of whom earned doctoral degrees. As my friend and colleague John E. Hall wrote, these achievements alone place Guyton among the greatest physiologists ever. So keep your brain and mind active by thinking and writing. I suggest starting with your life story. You are never too old to begin writing, and today marks an early age in the rest of your life.

3

The Aging Endocrine System

A Brief Introduction to Secretory Hormones

The classic definition of an endocrine hormone is a chemical compound that is produced by one organ or tissue and then transported by the blood to act on another organ or tissue. This definition has been modified in recent decades by new discoveries. For example, we now know that an endocrine hormone can act on cells or tissues in the vicinity of the producing or releasing cells. We call such an action a paracrine function of the hormone. Moreover, the same endocrine hormone can have an action on the very cells that produce and release it. This is called the autocrine function of the hormone. We now speak and write of autocrine, endocrine, and paracrine actions of hormones. In addition to past scientific breakthroughs related to the pancreas gland, insulin, and the treatment of diabetes, the field of physiology includes a more recent discovery: the connection between endocrinology, the kidneys, and elevated blood pressure.

The connection between renal ischemia and elevated blood pressure was first recognized at the beginning of the twentieth century. Patients with obstruction of renal blood flow (for example, congenital renal arterial stenosis and, later in life, diet-induced atherosclerosis) often had unexplained elevations in blood pressure. Investigators discovered that the kidneys produce a product called renin (pronounced rēnin). When renal blood flow is low (a condition called renal ischemia), renin is released into the systemic circulation. In the circulation, renin comes in contact with a large molecule produced by the liver that is called angiotensinogen. Acting enzymatically, renin clips off a small fragment of angiotensinogen. That smaller fragment is called angiotensin one (AI). When AI is exposed to another enzyme, it is reduced to angiotensin two (AII). AII is a potent vaso-constrictor. Its actions in the circulatory system led to increased arterial perfusion pressure and increased renal blood flow. The elevations in pres-sure and flow counteract the renal ischemia that triggered the release of renin, and a new steady state for kidney function is established. Thus, scientists discovered an endocrine-like role for the kidneys.

Now the field of endocrinology is aging. Approximately a hundred years ago, this branch of physiology was born after the discovery that in response to a stimulus, a tissue can release a chemical that is carried by the blood to a remote target, where it causes a response. Arguably, the near-simultaneous discovery and medical application of the three hor-mones secretin, gastrin, and insulin are chiefly responsible for the birth of endocrinology.

In 1902 the British physiologists William Bayliss and Ernest Starling were investigating the nervous system's control of digestion. It was already known that the pancreas secretes digestive juices in response to the pas-sage of food (chyme) into the proximal duodenum. The debate about whether locally released humorals (now called hormones, chemical mes-sengers, and so on) or the actions of peripheral nerves caused this secre-tion was heating up. By severing all nerves to the pancreas in experimental animals, Bayliss and Starling discovered that pancreatic secretory processes were not governed by the nervous system. They reasoned that a chemical substance, secreted by the small intestine, stimulates the pancreas after being transported there by the circulation. They named the substance secretin. Thus, secretin became the first chemical messenger or hormone discovered, and Bayliss coined the word "hormone" in 1905.

We now know that secretin is released into the intestinal lumen and systemic circulation in response to acidic duodenal pH and products of protein digestion. Secretin's main target is the pancreas, where it causes the excretion of a bicarbonate-rich fluid into the intestinal lumen. Bicarbonate ions buffer gastric acid and thus establish a pH favorable to the actions of other digestive enzymes in the small intestine. Ever since its discovery, secretin has been widely used in medicine as a test of pancreatic function. Its administration to a patient can provide valuable information about whether there are any abnormalities such as pancreatitis or pancreatic cancer.

Secretin is also found in neurons of the hypothalamus and along nerve tracts that descend into the posterior pituitary gland. These locations (particularly nuclei of the hypothalamus) suggest the involvement of secretin in osmoregulation, kidney function, and the homeostasis of body water (water found in various locations or compartments in the body—for example, intracellular water, interstitial water, and intravascular water such as that in the plasma). During periods of increased osmolality such as water restriction and excess thirst, secretin is released from the posterior pituitary. In the hypothalamus, secretin causes release of arginine vasopressin (AVP; also known as antidiuretic hormone, or ADH), a chemical messenger that helps conserve water by increasing its reabsorption in the kidneys. AVP is also needed to carry out the central effects of AII. Both AVP and AII are compounds involved in the regulation of body water and cardiovascular variables such as blood pressure and the effective volume of circulating blood. In experimental gene-knockout mice that are devoid of secretin, central injection of AII is unable to cause release of AVP and therefore cannot stimulate thirst or the intake of water.

Since the last decade of the twentieth century, the concept of translational medicine has been key to progress in the biomedical sciences. Translational medicine means rapidly transferring discoveries from research laboratories to the patient's bedside. In 1869 Paul Langerhans, then a medical student in Berlin, identified some previously undetected structures scattered throughout the pancreas. These small clusters of cells later became known as the islets of Langerhans. In the late nineteenth century European physicians and scientists, including Oscar Minkowski, working in collaboration with Joseph von Mering, removed the pancreas from healthy dogs to test its assumed role in digestion. Several days after the operation, Minkowski's technician noticed flies feeding on the dog's urine. When the scientists tested the urine, they found sugar in it— establishing for the first time a connection between the pancreas and diabetes. In 1901 the American physician and scientist Eugene Opie reported the link between the islets of Langerhans and diabetes: "Diabetes mellitus . . . is caused by destruction of the islets of Langerhans and occurs only when these bodies are in part or wholly destroyed."

During the next two decades, multiple attempts were made to isolate products of the islets as a potential treatment for diabetes. In 1906 George Ludwig Zuelzer was partially successful treating dogs with pancreatic extract but was unable to continue his work. Between 1911 and 1912 Ernest Lyman Scott at the University of Chicago used aqueous pancreatic extracts and noted a slight reduction in glucose in the urine. Unable to convince his supervisor of the work's value, he had to discontinue it. In 1915 Israel Kleiner, at Rockefeller University, demonstrated similar effects, but his work was interrupted by World War I and he did not return to it. In 1916 Nicolae Paulescu, a professor of physiology at the University of Medicine and Pharmacy in Bucharest, developed an aqueous pancreatic extract that, when injected into a diabetic dog, had a normalizing effect on circulating concentrations of blood sugar. He wrote four papers about his work before having to interrupt it because of World War I.

After the war Frederick Banting, a Canadian surgeon, read one of Minkowski's papers. He concluded that it was the very digestive secretions Minkowski had originally studied that were breaking down the islets' secretory products, thereby making it impossible to extract them. He reasoned that the internal secretions of the pancreas might hold the key to the treatment of diabetes. Banting knew that selected arteries could be tied off, causing most of the pancreas to atrophy while leaving the islets of Langerhans intact. He also knew that a relatively pure extract could be made from the islets once most of the rest of the pancreas was gone.

In the spring of 1921 Banting traveled to Toronto to explain his idea to J.J.R. Macleod, a professor of physiology at the University of Toronto. Banting asked Macleod if he could use his lab to test the idea. Macleod was initially skeptical but eventually agreed. For the experiments Macleod supplied Banting with ten dogs and offered him two medical students as laboratory assistants, Charles Best and Clark Noble. Banting needed only one assistant, so Best and Noble tossed a coin to see who would assist Banting. Best won and eventually shared half of Banting's portion of the Nobel Prize money and a large part of the credit for the discovery of insulin.

Banting's experimental method was to tie a ligature around the pancreatic duct. When the digestive cells of the pancreas were examined several weeks later, they had atrophied and been engulfed by the immune system, leaving thousands of islets. The investigators then isolated an extract from these islets, producing what they called isletin (now insulin). They tested their extract on dogs beginning in July 1921, and were able to keep a diabetic dog named Marjorie alive for the rest of the summer by injecting her with the crude extract they had prepared.

Banting and Best presented their results to Macleod on his return to Toronto in the fall of 1921, but Macleod found flaws in their experimental design and suggested repeating the experiments with more dogs and better equipment. He supplied the investigators with a better laboratory and, from his research grants, began paying Banting a salary. The experiments were repeated and after solving problems of extraction and purification, on January 11, 1922, Leonard Thompson, a fourteen-year-old diabetic who was dying at the Toronto General Hospital, was given the first injection of insulin. Unfortunately the extract was so impure that Thompson suffered a severe allergic reaction, and further injections were canceled. Over the next twelve days Banting, Best, and others worked day and night to improve the pancreatic extracts and Thompson was given a second dose on January 23. This time the outcome was near miraculous. Thompson started gaining weight and thrived physiologically. In less than a year, Banting's experimental methods in the dog laboratory were translated to diabetic patients and millions were being treated.

Prior to the discovery of insulin, children who were dying from diabetic ketoacidosis (acidic blood plasma caused by the metabolism of fatty acids in place of carbohydrates) were kept in large hospital wards of fifty or more patients. Most were unconscious. Helpless and grieving families often stood by, awaiting the inevitable death of their loved ones. During one of the monumental moments in modern medicine, Banting, Best, and others moved from bed to bed in one such ward, injecting the patients with newly purified insulin extract. To the joy and elation of their families, before Banting and Best reached the last dying children, the first were regaining consciousness.

During the spring of 1922, Best improved his extraction and purification techniques so that larger quantities of insulin could be produced on demand, even though the preparation remained impure. The drug manufacturer Eli Lilly and Company had offered assistance after the physiologists' first publications in 1921. In April 1922 the discoverers took Lilly up on the offer. By November Lilly had made a major breakthrough and was able to produce large quantities of highly refined insulin. Soon thereafter insulin was offered for sale around the world.

In the history of endocrinology a similar though less emotional story involves the discovery of gastrin and the intersection of the doctrines of nervism and the chemical regulation of stomach physiology. The doctrine of nervism was a twentieth-century notion that nerves do all regulating of physiological function. At that time the predominant ideas about the regulation of gastric secretory activity had been developed by the Russian neurophysiologist Ivan Petrovich Pavlov. Experiments on dogs in his laboratory had showed that the secretory behavior of gastric glands could be stimulated by a psychosomatic response via vagal innervation. Because this initial activity was transient, Pavlov proposed that later stages of the response might be controlled by excitatory substances acting on the sensory gastric nerves, thereby evoking increased glandular activity. Pavlov rejected the notion that the mechanism could involve excitatory chemicals delivered by the circulation rather than being released by nerves. It took only time and a few well-designed experiments to convince Pavlov and others of their mistaken notions.

Growth, Longevity, and the Aging Endocrine System

The main organs in the mammalian endocrine and neuroendocrine systems include the hypothalamus and its median eminence; the pituitary gland, with its stalk and anterior and posterior lobes; the adrenal glands, both cortex and medulla; the pancreas; the gonads; and the thyroid gland. There are other endocrine-like organs and tissues, but limitations of space preclude their discussion here (for example, the endocrine functions of the kidneys and cardiac atria). Considering all of these, one would be hard pressed to prove that endocrines are not involved in most body functions, including our physical and emotional states. For example, anxiety and depression are omnipresent in most societies. The body, brain, and mind are frequently exposed to challenges such as excessive or prolonged release of oxidants and pro-inflammatory chemicals that have the potential for lasting nerve and tissue damage. Our protection from these assaults comes, in part, from both the endocrine and the immune systems.

Our survival and well-being require us to continuously adapt to these external and internal challenges. These adaptations are achieved through

sensory signals integrated in the brain that lead to coordinated autonomic, behavioral, and endocrine responses that sustain homeostasis.
Fortunately, there are intrinsic defense mechanisms that protect neuroendocrine tissue and other cells against such damage. Decreasing regulatory
ability and other alterations of these protective mechanisms during aging
result in reduced neuroendocrine resilience to challenges and is con-
ducive to neuronal and endocrine damage. Evidence from animal and
human studies indicates that diminishing activity of the adrenal and pituitary glands, as well as of the hypothalamus, contributes to the physiology
of aging. One example is the circulating concentrations of glucocorticoids
and their age-dependent changes.

Circulating concentrations of glucocorticoids (stress hormones)
depend, in part, on the activity of the hypothalamus-pituitary-adrenal
axis, but there is not always a correlation between plasma corticosteroids
and adrenocorticotropic hormone in humans. Some studies have found
that aging is associated with elevated basal concentrations of glucocorticoids in the morning, but others have found a loss of diurnal rhythmicity
of glucocorticoids in aging humans. Moreover, the corticosterone
response to acute stress and lifetime changes in the steroid hormones
released from the adrenal cortex (adrenocorticosteroids) vary across individuals. About 40 percent of older adults display a marked increase in
these hormones, a similar proportion show a modest increase, and the
remaining 20 percent reveal a decrease in cortisol as they age. The differences are likely to be genetically determined, as shown by studies of twins
and by differences found between strains of laboratory animals.

Hyperactivity of the hypothalamus-pituitary-adrenal axis contributes
to neuronal and peripheral deterioration during aging. Thus, an inability
to limit chronic stress probably increases the effects of aging due to prolonged exposure to stress hormones. Conversely, those who practice activities that reduce stress appear to age more gracefully than those who don't.
Practices such as yoga, avoiding negativity and pessimism, and meditating
regularly have all been said to reduce chronic stress and to improve health
and well-being. The major neuroendocrine response to stress involves
neurons of specific nuclei in the hypothalamus such as the paraventricular nucleus, and the release of their secretory products such as neuro-
peptides, corticotrophin-releasing hormone, and AVP. Such secretory

products stimulate the release of pituitary adrenocorticotropic hormone, which, in turn, augments secretion of glucocorticoids by the adrenal cortex. The augmented release of the glucocorticoids is essential to one's ability to adapt to stress.

Glucocorticoids such as cortisol in humans and corticosterone in experimental rodents act on specific receptors in most tissues, including the brain, by initiating circulatory, metabolic, and neuromodulatory changes that are appropriate responses to the challenges of stress. In addition to increased release of adrenocorticotropic hormone and other glucocorticoids, the hypothalamic peptides AVP and corticotropin-releasing hormone are released in the brain, where they mediate behavioral and autonomic responses to stress. Thus it is clear that acute activation of the hypothalamus-pituitary-adrenal axis is necessary for one's adaptations to the stressors of life. Conversely, sustained elevations in circulating concentrations of stress hormones can predispose one to cardiovascular, immune, metabolic, psychiatric, and reproductive disorders. This is seen in both humans and experimental animals.

Appropriate and timely termination of one's response to stress is essential to physiological harmony throughout the life span. The inability to limit one's response to chronic stress is likely to enhance the effects of aging due to the pathophysiological consequences of prolonged exposure to stress hormones. Also, depressed people are at increased risk of developing physical illnesses commonly seen with aging, and chronic and inescapable early-life adversities can lead, with age, to depression and related medical comorbidities.

Growth and longevity are fundamental components of aging. Both are affected by our attitudes toward calories, diet, and nutrition. In virtually all organisms, life expectancy is profoundly affected by caloric intake. As discussed in previous chapters, most studies have found that consuming fewer calories without causing malnourishment lengthens life. Eating to excess shortens it. Findings in invertebrates indicate that metabolic-sensing neurons detect changes in caloric intake and send signals throughout the body to indicate a variation in energy status. The mammalian hypothalamus contains neurons that detect variations in normal energy balance and the homeostasis of carbohydrate and lipid metabolism. For example, some of these neurons are known to suppress or increase body weight and to be critical regulators of glucose homeostasis. Defects in them lead to increased body fat, insulin resistance, and the metabolic syndrome, all of which are typical age-related disorders.

Some scientists have suggested that members of the sirtuins family of proteins regulate longevity at the molecular level. Sirtuins (SIRT, or silent information regulators) are enzymes that regulate the expression of genes and cellular function. There are seven members of the mammalian family of SIRT proteins (SIRT1–7). The founding member is SIRT-2. Due in part to their dependence on nicotinamide adenine dinucleotide, sirtuins are thought to be molecular links between dietary restriction and longevity. In support of this theory, knocking out the SIRT-2 gene in fruit flies reduces diet-restricted longevity, and overexpression of SIRT-2 extends flies' life span. In mice the increase in ambulation caused by restricting calories requires SIRT-1. SIRT-1 is abundantly expressed in metabolic-sensing neurons of the hypothalamus, and these neurons control insulin sensitivity in liver and muscle, as well as the content of brown adipose tissue in visceral fat—that is, fat that is integral to abdominal organs such as the gut, the liver, and pancreas and to internal reproductive organs.

Such experimental observations in animals predict that hypothalamic sirtuins are involved in regulating the metabolic aging process in all peripheral organs. As such, they are in a position to influence circulating concentrations of the products of adipocytes, hepatocytes, and myocytes, which ultimately contribute to changes in health and longevity. Hypothalamic neurons control other physiological variables that are known to deteriorate with age. Hypothalamic neurons have been shown to influence the liver's sensitivity to insulin via the vagus nerve, whereas neurons of the ventromedial hypothalamus help coordinate the sensitivity to insulin of the skeletal muscle.

Prominent age-associated adaptations in the secretion of gonadal products such as luteinizing hormone, testosterone, and somatotropin (growth hormone) are predictable in humans. Consider, for example, the television advertisements for low testosterone in aging men that were not seen prior to about 2013. Low testosterone has attracted considerable public attention since the early days of erectile dysfunction, when drug companies discovered how lucrative the sales of Viagra, Cialis, and Levitra were. With age the symptoms in men of low circulating concentrations of testosterone and other androgens include but are not limited to muscle weakness, muscle wasting, diminished physical stamina, erectile dysfunction, systolic hypertension, thickness of the carotid artery wall, abdominal visceral-fat mass, insulin resistance, low concentrations of high density lipoproteins (HDLs), drowsiness after eating, impaired quality of life, depressive mood, diminished working memory, decreased executive-cognitive function, reduced strength of grip, decreased lean-body mass, and increased visceral fat. These same symptoms are significantly reversed by administration of testosterone.

A fifteen-year prospective study conducted in New Mexico revealed that total testosterone concentrations fall by approximately 110 nanograms per deciliter per decade in men ages sixty and older. The Massachusetts Male Aging Cohort study and the Baltimore Longitudinal Study of Aging have reported similar and related findings. Transdermal administration of five milligrams of testosterone daily, combined with subcutaneous growth hormone at about six micrograms per kilogram body weight per day for one month in older men increases the expression of muscle insulin-like growth-factor-I gene, levels of insulin-like growth factor I, lean body mass, measures of physical performance, levels of growth hormone, and osteocalcin concentrations.

Somatotropin—also known as growth hormone, as mentioned above—increases the production and release of insulin-like growth factors and their binding proteins in target tissues such as skeletal muscle; it also promotes growth. The hormone stimulates the breakdown of fat and the proliferation of cartilage and growth of precursors to red blood cells. It also produces insulin-like growth factors in the brain. Among other things, this enhances the growth of spines on nerve cell bodies, formation of synapses, differentiation of neurons, and stability of memory. Of the roughly 2,000 genes in the human liver, more than 850 occur only in males and more than 750 only in females, due to strong dependence on the pulse patterns defined by growth hormone.

Continuous administration of growth hormone releasing factors for one month elevates circulating concentrations of growth hormone, insulin-like growth factor I, and its binding proteins in middle-aged adults. Treating patients two times each day for thirty days also improves their ability to climb stairs and to take short walks. Such drug treatments also reduce the content of fat in abdominal organs and increase lean body mass. Thus, it seems possible to attenuate or slow the effects of aging by administering selected endocrine hormones that are known to influence growth and development. As good as all this sounds, you will notice that there is no mention of side effects here. Moreover, this is such new therapy that no one knows what to expect after a year of administration of testosterone, let alone after five years or more. Arguably, getting thirty to sixty minutes of physical activity each day will do the same or even more for muscle mass, endurance, strength, and other markers of low testosterone. Moreover, what did we learn about hormone replacement therapy in women after five to ten years of experience?

The Aging Pituitary Gland

The pituitary gland is interposed between the hypothalamus and peripheral endocrine organs (for example, the adrenal glands and gonads). Other endocrine organs such as the thyroid gland and pancreas are also influenced by the pituitary. The human pituitary is really two glands in one: the anterior pituitary gland (the anterior lobe) and the posterior pituitary gland (the posterior lobe). The anterior lobe is also known as the adenohypophysis and the posterior lobe as the neurohypophysis. The pituitary is also called the hypophyseal gland. The anterior lobe is the site of synthesis, storage, and release of the following hormones: adrenocorticotropic hormone, follicle-stimulating hormone, leutinizing hormone, thyroid-stimulating hormone (TSH), growth hormone, and prolactin. The posterior lobe does not synthesize hormones, but stores and releases two of them: oxytocin and AVP. These hormones are synthesized by large neurons whose cell bodies are found in the paraventricular and supraoptic nuclei of the hypothalamus. Oxytocin and AVP are then transported down the axons of these neurons, through the median eminence and pituitary stalk (which attaches the pituitary to the hypothalamus and its median eminence), and into the posterior pituitary, where—like neurotransmitters—they are stored for later release. AVP is synthesized and released in response to hyperosmolality (excess salinity) of the extracellular water near its corresponding hypothalamic nuclei. Oxytocin is regulated and released during childbirth and lactation.

The supraoptic nucleus is located above the optic nerve tract. This suggested to early investigators that the supraoptic nucleus was involved in vision and its regulation. However, research in the early 1960s showed that after surgical or chemical removal of the supraoptic nucleus, the optic nerves of experimental animals remained intact and did not atrophy because of disuse. Three decades later, electrophysiological studies indicated the presence of an input from the optic nerve to the supraoptic nucleus in rodents, but it is still not known whether such an input exists in humans. The major endocrine products of the supraoptic nucleus—AVP and oxytocin—act both as neuroendocrines and as neurotransmitters in the brain and are involved in a great number of different physiological functions. They are both neuromodulators.

Secretion of AVP is activated by osmotic stimuli, low circulating blood volume (hypovolemia), low blood pressure (hypotension), liver glycogenolysis, and hypoglycemia (low circulating concentrations of blood glucose). AVP is released into the portal microcirculation of the pituitary stalk and also participates in the secretion of corticosteroids during stress and trauma. AVP is also involved in the regulation of body temperature (thermoregulation), blood pressure and tissue perfusion (vasoconstrictor responses), brain development, circadian rhythms, maintenance of memory, and aggression and paternal behavior. AVP is also released during sexual arousal and in the stress of labor and parturition.

Because of the central role of AVP in the regulation of body water and its distribution, and because of the frequent disturbances of water and electrolyte balance in the elderly, there has been increasing interest during the last decade or so in the physiology of the aging posterior pituitary gland. However, data on changes in the secretion of AVP and thirst drive in the elderly are still lacking. Most studies of circulating concentrations of AVP report that they are higher in elderly than in younger subjects. The number of neurons expressing AVP in the paraventricular nucleus, but not in the supraoptic nucleus, increases with age. Neither seems to be affected by dementias such as Alzheimer's disease.

Pathophysiological activity of secretory neurons can often be surmised by examining their subcellular structures. In part, aging in both the supraoptic and paraventricular nuclei can be determined from the increase in size of nucleoli and the Golgi apparatus. This information can be complemented by measurements of the enhanced circulating plasma concentrations of vasopressin and simultaneously released products such as neurophysins. Moreover, age-dependent hyperactivity of vasopressin-expressing neurons in the hypothalamus appears to be gender related. In men younger than fifty, the sizes of vasopressin-expressing neurons and their Golgi apparatus, as well as the contents of messenger-RNA in both the supraoptic and paraventricular nuclei, were greater than in women of corresponding ages. These differences in young people according to gender is in agreement with the higher plasma concentrations of AVP found in men compared with women, even though the secretory activity of these neurons does not change significantly with aging in men. As women age and enter the peri- and postmenopausal states, these same measures of supraoptic and paraventricular secretory activity increase, when compared with the measures in younger women. Thus it appears that aging-related increases in AVP occur primarily in women.

When compared to older men and young women, increased activity of AVP-releasing neurons in young men and elderly women is accompanied by higher simultaneous expression of estrogen receptors. In young women, who have the lowest secretory activity for AVP, estrogen receptors were found in the AVP neurons to a considerably larger extent than in men and postmenopausal women. This suggests an inhibitory activity of estrogen on these neurons in younger women. In addition, expression of the neurotrophin receptor (the binding site for nerve growth factors) was enhanced in the supraoptic nucleus in postmenopausal women, compared with its expression in younger women. This implicates neurotrophins and their receptors in postmenopausal activation of AVP-expressing neurons. It also suggests a possible interaction between estrogens, neurotrophins, and their receptors in the regulation of AVP neuronal activity. Since estrogens inhibit the expression of neurotrophin receptors, estrogens would also appear to reduce the secretory effects of neurotrophins on AVP-releasing neurons, resulting in smaller size of cells, smaller size of the Golgi apparatus, and lower production of AVP messenger-RNA in young women.

The roles of oxytocin in the physiology of lactation and parturition are well documented, but its central functions—such as the facilitation of maternal behavior, lordosis, and inhibition of learning and memory—are less well understood. Oxytocin has been shown to be released at the time of ejaculation, and circulating plasma concentrations of the hormone are significantly increased during sexual arousal in both men and women. Oxytocin has been implicated in eating disorders, and both AVP and oxytocin are important in social attachment. Little is known about the effects of aging in humans on these activities.

The physiological relationships among the hypothalamus, pituitary, and gonads are called the hypothalamic-pituitary-gonadal (HPG) axis. This axis has been intensely investigated. Gonadotropin-releasing hormone (GnRH, produced in the hypothalamus) has been historically thought of as a neuroendocrine hormone or factor that stimulates release of the gonadal hormones—follicle-stimulating hormone and leutinizing hormone—from the anterior pituitary. Both hormones target reproductive tissues in the testes, ovaries, and other peripheral organs. Only recently has GnRH been thought of as a centrally acting hormone. Evidence is mounting that GnRH has multiple sites of action in both the male and female central nervous systems, specifically the cerebrum, hypothalamus, and brainstem.

GnRH plays a vital role in both the central and peripheral regulation of reproduction. GnRH-like compounds and receptors of GnRH are found throughout the brain, where they are thought to influence psychosomatic and cognitive functions, eating behavior, intelligence, learning, and memory. Epidemiological support is suggested by a reduction in neurodegenerative disease after therapy with agonists of GnRH. Changes in circulating and neuronal concentrations of the hormones of the HPG axis (for example, increased gonadotropins, increased GnRH, and decreased reproductive steroids) after menopause or andropause can profoundly alter the behavior of neurons. Experimentally modifying the GnRH-mediated release of leutinizing hormone promotes cellular and molecular changes that are similar to neurodegenerative findings in Alzheimer's disease. Moreover, women who maintain relatively high levels of endogenous estrogen and functional HPG axes after menopause exhibit a decreased prevalence of Alzheimer's disease.

Benefits of hormone replacement therapy, however, suggest that the declining concentrations of steroid hormones that accompany menopause or andropause cannot adequately explain susceptibility to dementia. In fact, it is only when we take into account the roles of other hormones and receptor systems of the HPG axis that we can accurately characterize the susceptibility to and onset and progression of dementia (for example, GnRH can affect the function of the hippocampus and cerebral cortex during a critical period around menopause or andropause). Such observations suggest that therapies based on GnRH receptors could be useful in treating dementia, and controlled clinical trials are under way to test this hypothesis.

Hormonal systems other than the HPG axis have recently been implicated in aging as well. For example, the central melanocortin system is defined as a collection of circuits in the central nervous system that express proteins having orexigenic and anorexigenic properties (properties related to eating disorders). The system originates in the hypothalamus and includes downstream targets that express melanocortin-3 and melanocortin-4 receptors. The central melanocortin system seems to be crucial for normal energy balance in humans and rodents, and we know that blood sugars, amino acids, fatty acids, and many hormones help regulate energy homeostasis. It is equally clear that the central melanocortin system, meant to decrease energy intake in times of surplus, ultimately fails in obese subjects. Human patients with central melanocortin mutations are obese (as are gene-knockout mice designed to permit research on this system).

The central melanocortin system is involved in the regulation of body weight through its role in appetite and energy expenditure via the recently discovered compounds leptin, ghrelin, and agouti-related protein. The system receives input from hormones, nutrients, and afferent sensory neurons, and it is unique in its composition of neurons that express both agonists and antagonists of melanocortin receptors. For example, stimulation of the melanocortin-4 receptor causes a decrease in appetite as well as an increase in metabolism in fat and muscle cells even in a relatively starved state. Damage to this receptor causes moribund obesity. Because of the obesity pandemic, the central melanocortin system is an increasing target for drugs that treat obesity, diabetes, and cardiovascular disease—all symptoms common in modern, high-tech societies.

The Aging Adrenal Cortex

In humans the adrenal glands are located bilaterally and atop the kidneys. Each of the glands has an adrenal capsule, an outer cortex, and an inner medulla. The cortex is divisible into three or four well-defined zones, each associated with the production of a different class of adrenal hormones. The products of the adrenal cortex that are released by the adrenocorticotropic hormone (so named because its target is the adrenal cortex) of the anterior pituitary are classified into three groups: glucocorticoids, mineralocorticoids, and sex steroids. Glucocorticoids are involved in the body's use of energy substrates, specifically carbohydrates such as glucose but also fat and protein. Mineralocorticoids play critical roles in the regulation and actions of electrolytes such as calcium, potassium, and sodium ions. And sex steroids target the reproductive organs and related tissues. The sex steriods include the androgens, estrogens, and progestins that are released by gonadal tissues.

Aging is arguably the most universal contributor to the causes of metabolic decline and related diseases such as metabolic syndrome and type II diabetes. Obesity complicates and amplifies these effects of aging. Insulin resistance represents a major component of the metabolic syndrome and is commonly observed in older adults. Major impairments include the unrestrained synthesis of glucose and other sugars by the liver, synthesis of lipids in fat cells, and defects in the synthesis of glycogen and uptake of glucose in skeletal muscle. Abdominal obesity, commonly observed with aging, is a major contributor to insulin resistance and metabolic syndrome. Many older people who have a normal body mass index (one's weight expressed in kilograms divided by one's height expressed in meters squared) display abdominal obesity, a factor that can decrease the usefulness of body mass index as a predictor of type II diabetes in older people. Aging is also associated with an increase in the pro-inflammatory cytokines that are known to interfere with the physiological actions of insulin. These cytokines are derived from both the age-associated accumulation of visceral fat and the secretion by increasing numbers of aging cells. Collectively, such age-related alterations in metabolism and distribution of body fat are active participants in a vicious cycle that accelerates the aging process and the onset of disease.

Sadly, few investigations have focused on aging-related changes that affect the different zones of the adrenal cortex. To help fill this void, one group of pathologists examined the adrenal glands of sixty-one patients who had died at ages ranging from one day to ninety-two years. These patients had no indication of primary adrenal disease, although in some there was evidence of stress-filled lives. In the youngest patients, the zona glomerulosa was well developed. Columns of cells projecting from the base of the cortex to the adrenal capsule could easily be discerned. After age forty, however, the zona glomerulosa occupied less than one-quarter of the adrenal circumference, revealing atrophy and degeneration in early middle age. This age-related remodeling featured changes that were based on the steroid products and enzymes that the cells expressed. The deeper subcortical tissues were occupied by a progenitor zone that expressed neither aldosterone- nor sex steroid–producing enzymes. These investigators hypothesized that atrophy of the zona glomerulosa and development of the progenitor zone might be related to the high-sodium and low-potassium diets common in human beings today.

Both AII and plasma potassium directly stimulate the zona glomerulosa to produce aldosterone. Moreover, AII is stimulated or suppressed by low or high dietary sodium, respectively, in a physiological feedback mechanism that is one of the pillars of the long-term regulation of blood pressure. Thus, the results of the pathologists' investigation just described are complementary to the established correlation between the incidence of age-related high blood pressure and excessive ingestion of salt. The daily intake of salt for the average man and woman, respectively, has been estimated as ten and seven grams per day in the United States, and twelve and ten grams per day in Japan. High intake of dietary salt suppresses the physiological renin-angiotensin system, and the comparatively low intake of dietary potassium fails to stimulate the adrenal cortex. The latter contributes to the atrophy of the adrenal glands and the corresponding elevations in blood pressure with age.

Other pathophysiological problems beset the adrenal cortex, and these can be seen as early as childhood and can last a lifetime. For example, seventy-eight otherwise healthy five- and six-year-old kindergarten children were studied to examine associations among stress-induced adversity (a phenomenon affecting the adrenal glands), autonomic nerves, and the lengths of telomeres in their cells. Parents provided consent and demographic information, while teachers and parents reported children's behavioral problems that were self-imposed or that originated from external sources (such as taunting by other children).

Cells from the children's mouths and the children's reactions to stress were studied in the spring of the kindergarten year.

Secretion of cortisol in the saliva (adrenocortical function), heart rate, and respiratory sinus arrhythmia (autonomic nerve function) were measured in response to standardized laboratory challenges. Respiratory sinus arrhythmia means that the respiratory cycle importantly and predictably affects cardiovascular functions such as heart rate and blood pressure. Typically, heart rate increases during inspiration and decreases during expiration. Such changes are caused by autonomic reflexes whose descriptions are beyond the scope of this book. These measures of children's health and responses to adversity were normalized for age, race, and gender. The investigators found that heart rate and cortisol concentrations were inversely related to the length of telomeres, but respiratory sinus arrhythmia was unrelated. The lengths of telomeres in children with high sympathetic activation and high parasympathetic withdrawal (decreasing respiratory sinus arrhythmia) did not differ. However, children with both this profile and elevated reactivity to stress (increased release of cortisol) had significantly shorter telomeres.

Findings like these suggest that psychosomatic processes can induce the early onset of aging, and that the length of telomeres might be helpful in identifying this (as discussed in chapter 1). The association of a child's reactivity to social stress and adversity with the length of telomeres from cells of the child's mouth suggest that children with greater sensitivity might prove to be more susceptible to aging-related physiological changes. The length of telomeres in a child's mouth might also serve as a marker of health in general, although more data are needed to establish the clinical significance of this speculation and its potential relationship to health in adulthood. Moreover, the mechanisms by which social adversity in childhood or at any other age contributes to the attrition of telomeres as well as to their lengths are unknown.

Early in life there is a rapid shortening of the telomeres in leukocytes, with greater decrements than during any other period in the human life cycle. The fact that adverse events early in life correlate with poorer health throughout life reveals how critical it is for children to grow up in environments that are physically and socially healthy. In adults, chronic adversity and greater perceptions of stress contribute to the shortening of telomeres. Again, the physiological mechanisms are unknown, but they might involve increased exposure to adrenocorticotropic hormones. More work is needed in this area.

In the offspring of animals that are administered excessive glucocorticoids or that are malnourished, permanent changes in behavioral, cardiovascular, metabolic, and neuroendocrine functions are seen. These seem to be mediated, in part, by changes in the metabolism of glucocorticoids. Exposure to extreme malnutrition or stress during critical periods of prenatal or postnatal development is associated with long-lasting changes in the psychosomatic and physiological well-being of individuals in adulthood. Most studies have emphasized the detrimental effects of excess exposure to stress hormones. However, scientists are increasingly recognizing that some consequences of extreme stress are advantageous, and that there appear to be critical developmental windows for such effects.

As examples, consider the following. Adult offspring of women who were pregnant in Holland during the winter of 1944–45 (called the Dutch Hunger Winter) and thus exposed to stress show increased rates of cardiovascular disease and schizophrenia if during that winter their mothers were in the first trimester of pregnancy but decreased glucose intolerance if their mothers were in the third trimester. Women who developed posttraumatic stress disorder by being in or near New York's World Trade Center on 9/11 during pregnancy are another example. Their offspring had reduced concentrations of salivary cortisol if on 9/11 their mothers were in the last trimester of pregnancy. Extreme malnutrition and related adversity during development are associated with long-lasting alterations in the metabolism of glucocorticoids. These effects might be adaptive and could lead to lower risks of cardiovascular, metabolic, and stress-related disorders later in life.

Findings such as these suggest that the developmental timing during which adversity occurs might define the nature of persistent outcomes. For example, survivors of the Holocaust showed reductions in cortisol, 5α-tetrahydrocortisol, and enhanced production of total glucocorticoids. The elevation in total glucocorticoids was associated with lower enzymatic degradation of cortisol. The greatest decrements in cortisol were associated with the earliest ages of exposure to the Holocaust and less severe symptoms following the Holocaust. Cardiovascular and metabolic manifestations of cardiovascular and metabolic abnormalities in survivors were also associated with decreased enzymatic activity.

The Aging Adrenal Medulla

In considering the aging adrenal medulla, it is helpful to think of the aging response to catecholamines such as epinephrine and norepinephrine (adrenalin and noradrenalin). Both the adrenal medulla and sympathetic nerves release norepinephrine, epinephrine, and related compounds in response to stress and other stimuli. When he published his theory of the fight-or-flight response, Walter Cannon became the first to describe hormones as biomarkers of stress. Cannon was thinking of immediate versus delayed physiological reactions when he considered the response to pending danger of a human or other animal. His experimental results led him to conclude that fight-or-flight responses begin with activation of the sympathetic nervous system. Stress-induced activation of this branch of the autonomic nervous system, Cannon reasoned, stimulates the release of epinephrine and norepinephrine. The response includes shifting systemic arterial blood flow away from temporarily less important organs (such as the gastrointestinal tract, skin, and kidneys) to organs more vital to either fight or flight (including the adrenal glands, brain, heart, and skeletal muscle).

Today, fluid concentrations of epinephrine and norepinephrine are among the premier physiological markers of stimulated sympathetic nerves and adrenal medulla. These products of stress and anxiety are routinely measured in blood plasma, urine, and cerebrospinal fluid. Circulating epinephrine, norepinephrine, and related metabolites are rapidly metabolized, but elevated levels of them indicate immediate changes in the activation of sympathetic nerves and adrenal medulla. The complications of withdrawing and sampling blood, as well as the short half-life of catecholamines, make it difficult if not impossible to monitor circulating plasma concentrations of catecholamines outside the laboratory. Happily, analysis of urine provides a relatively noninvasive method of measurement, and the collection of urine at home by patients and experimental subjects has been used successfully in studies of chronic stress. Of course, one must take into consideration the lag time (a matter of hours) between the onset of stress and anxiety and the appearance of such chemicals in the urine.

Due, in part, to physiological deterioration of sympathetic nerves and adrenal medulla, a variety of age-related changes occur in the cardiovascular and other organ systems. For example, both pulmonary and systemic arterial blood pressures gradually increase until one reaches approximately seventy years of age. Then systolic and diastolic arterial pressures begin to plateau. The baseline resting heart rate remains relatively constant throughout adulthood, whereas exercise-induced maximum heart rate gradually decreases with age. For a competitive athlete, this can be disappointing. A runner, swimmer, or dancer might have used maximal heart rate for years as one indicator of physical fitness. As this number declines, it is an indication of the effects of aging on a body. It is akin to lying on the weight bench at age sixty and realizing that you can no longer safely do the fifty-pound butterflies that you did at an earlier age.

In older age, response to acute stress or extra physical activity is associated with marked elevations in systolic blood pressure, whereas diastolic pressure rises more moderately. In contrast, the elevations in heart rate (tachycardia) associated with physical activity and psychosocial stress are attenuated in older individuals. Moreover, aging is associated with higher concentrations of norepinephrine in circulating plasma. This could be due to aging-related increments in the release of norepinephrine, reduced metabolic clearance of the neurotransmitter, (clearance is the removal of a compound from the circulation, usually by the kidneys and/or the liver) or a combination of the two in older adults. In contrast, basal release of epinephrine from the adrenal medulla declines in older age. This is not always accompanied by reduced circulating concentrations of epinephrine, however, because of impaired clearance. In addition, the diurnal increase in norepinephrine is attenuated from young adulthood to midlife.

Notwithstanding what I have said above about the aging adrenal cortex, the sympathoadrenal medullary axis (the coordinated action of the sympathetic nervous system and adrenal medulla) is the body's primary physiological response to acute stressors. Following a bout of acute stress, norepinephrine impedes digestion and gastrointestinal motility, increases circulating concentrations of plasma glucose, and dilates the pupils. Correspondingly, both norepinephrine and epinephrine increase heart rate and cardiac contractility (blood flow to organs and tissues), relax visceral and vascular smooth muscle (reduces resistance to blood flow), and increase the release of glucose from stores such as the liver (glycogenolysis). The rise in circulating catecholamines depends on the type and magnitude of the stressor: it doubles their resting levels during routine daily activities and doubles that when moderately severe stressors are imposed (for example, in athletic competitions).

Other important determinants of the reactivity of the sympathoadrenal medullary axis are the characteristics of the stressor, such as whether it can be controlled, whether it causes fear or anger, and whether it is likely to be accompanied by pleasure and pain. As stressors increase over time, the frequency and duration of sympathetic discharge also increase, possibly resulting in tissue damage. For example, if a vasoconstrictor response is too severe or lasts too long, tissue ischemia (insufficient blood flow and oxygen delivery) and even necrosis (tissue death) can occur. Severe acute stressors can alter electrophysiological properties of cells leading, in some cases, to cardiac arrhythmias. There are reports of people—not just elderly ones—who have been startled to death by sudden, unexpected stress (for example, the explosion in a natural gas line in Edison, New Jersey, in March 1994).

The Aging Thyroid

Dysfunction of the thyroid gland in aging adults is prevalent in industrialized societies and can be associated with significant morbidity and mortality if left untreated. The reasons a malfunctioning thyroid might not be treated are multiple and include minimal symptoms when a patient is being examined and the likelihood of harm from treatment (such as overdosing a patient with a hypoactive thyroid). Also, a person's physiological state can predispose him or her to adverse reactions from synthetic thyroid analogs and related treatments. Moreover, differences in thyroid function, the production and release of TSH by the pituitary, dietary intake of iodine, and the presence of autoimmune thyroid disease obscure the distinction of age- and disease-related thyroid abnormalities. Finally, interpreting the results of tests of thyroid function can be challenging for clinicians because of a patient's chronic illness, excess consumption of medications by the aging, and related age-dependent physiological changes.

The classic symptoms of both hypo- and hyperthyroidism can be absent in patients with thyroid dysfunction—or overlooked in older patients—making the diagnosis and treatment even more difficult. Whether antithyroid antibody is present or not, investigators have reported both increased and decreased circulating concentrations of plasma TSH with increasing age. Despite this confusion, the prevailing evidence suggests that as one ages, circulating plasma concentrations of TSH rise. For example, one group of investigators found plasma concentrations of TSH to be significantly higher in an older group (with an average age of ninety-eight years) than in a younger control group. Several other studies have reported increased TSH levels (with eighty-five years as the average age of subjects) and low to normal thyroxine concentrations (with the subjects' average age seventy-eight years) to be associated with improved longevity in older adults.

Such findings make some sense, at least among the elderly who do not overeat. Often older people lose their appetite for food as they age. Disinterest in food and other necessities of life can be precipitated by factors such as the death of a spouse or being institutionalized against one's will. If an elderly person is malnourished and simultaneously has sustained elevated thyroxine concentrations, one result will be a loss of weight and failure to thrive. And although data on possible mechanisms for this effect in older adults are still lacking, the correlation between higher levels of TSH and longevity is hypothesized to be due to reduced bioavailability of thyroxine and attenuated metabolism. Moreover, the adult children (average age of seventy years) of individuals showing familial longevity also have elevated circulating concentrations of TSH, indicating a genetic element to the finding. Still, the management of thyroid disorders in older adults remains controversial, and current guidelines suggest choosing treatment on an individual basis.

About twenty-five years ago my wife was diagnosed with hypothyroidism. A small benign nodule was found on her thyroid gland and was surgically removed, and she was placed on a synthetic thyroid drug. Her endocrinologists were never able to determine the appropriate dose. While she was taking the drug, my wife was restless, sleep-deprived, and on edge much of the time. After a couple years of unsuccessful professional help, she reduced her daily dose by about 50 percent. By the end of another

year, her drug-related symptoms had not changed. She decided to stop taking the drug altogether. Within a few months her restlessness, sleepless
nights, and elevated body temperature had subsided, and life for her
returned to normal. The drug did not work for her. It has been more than
twenty years since she discontinued taking the drug, and she continues to
monitor her TSH and thyroxine levels with annual physical exams and corresponding blood work. Neither she nor her current physician finds any
reasons for thyroid-related concerns.

Hyperthyroidism in older adults is estimated to be as high as 4 percent
in the United States, with Graves' disease being the most common form.
The prevalence of both multinodular goiter and cancer of the thyroid
increases with age. Two-thirds of older adults with hyperthyroidism have
symptoms of sympathetic overactivity, tremors, anxiety, palpitations, loss
of weight, and inability to tolerate heat. Symptoms are similar in younger
patients. However, one-third of patients age seventy and older see their
physicians with loss of weight, shortness of breath, ventricular tachycardia, and indifference to their condition (apathetic hyperthyroidism). More
common is subclinical hyperthyroidism, which has a prevalence of 8 percent and is more common in women than men, especially in patients over
the age of seventy. Women sixty years of age or older with this condition
usually do not develop overt hyperthyroidism as they age: fewer than
1 percent per year make this transition.

Age is independently associated with an increased risk of developing
atrial fibrillation in both men and women. Atrial fibrillation is estimated
to be present in 20–35 percent of older patients suffering from hyperthyroidism. It is especially common in those with diseased nodules on their
thyroid glands. In older patients, sustained reductions in circulating
plasma concentrations of TSH are associated with a threefold increase
in the risk of developing atrial fibrillation. Also, because of a greater
incidence of underlying cardiac disease in patients over age sixty, the
risk of developing atrial fibrillation increases with age. Moreover, atrial
fibrillation in aging adults might sometimes be the only clinical sign of
hyperthyroidism.

As we age, all soft tissues atrophy. This includes the cardiac pacemaker or sinoatrial node and the specialized cardiac conduction system
that connects the node with atrial and ventricular tissues (muscle, nerves,

and connective tissue). Degeneration of the node with age and corresponding fibrotic changes in the conduction system make the occurrence of
palpitations less likely. In contrast, younger patients suffering from hyperthyroidism often have sinus tachycardia or elevated heart rates. This is
physiologically problematic because the longer the heart beats at a faster
rate, the more work it does. More cardiac work requires more coronary
blood flow and a greater supply of oxygen. But if one has chronic atherosclerosis of the coronary arteries (an age-related condition that occurs in
many elderly people), the supply of blood and oxygen to the heart is
already compromised. This can make elevations in cardiac work dangerous and even fatal.

Overt hyperthyroidism can also be accompanied by elevated differences in systolic and diastolic blood pressures (jointly called pulse pressure), inability to perform physical activity, increased risk for atrial
fibrillation, and ventricular hypertrophy (increased mass of cardiac tissue). Elevations in pulse pressure are often caused by increased systolic
blood pressure and not by decreased diastolic pressure with constant systolic pressure. Such changes in systolic blood pressure correspondingly
increase cardiac work and place additional stress on the heart. Several
studies have found that decreased plasma concentrations of TSH are
accompanied by increased cardiovascular mortality in the elderly. As mentioned above, subclinical hyperthyroidism is associated with ventricular
hypertrophy, which is an ominous predictor of cardiovascular mortality.

In older women, hyperthyroidism is a well-recognized risk factor for
low mineral density in bones and for bone fractures. Thyroid hormones act
on matrix-forming bone cells to increase the release of calcium, thus leading to a net loss of bone density with age. Notably, most studies that have
documented the relationship between dysfunctional thyroid glands and
fractures of bones have been done in women. In one large study, investigators reported that women over the age of sixty-five with low plasma
concentrations of TSH had a three- to fourfold increased risk for hip and
vertebral fractures when compared with control subjects having normal
concentrations of plasma TSH.

The incidence of hypothyroidism steadily increases with advancing
age, predominantly due to the rising prevalence of autoimmune diseases
such as Hashimoto's disease (or autoimmune thyroiditis). In one survey,

the incidence of Hashimoto's disease was 67 percent among subjects with an average age of seventy-three years. A study of endocrinologists' patients revealed that 47 percent of them age fifty-five years and older received a diagnosis of autoimmune thyroid disease. Only 37 percent had hypothyroidism from other causes (such as a surgical overdose of radioiodine). Moreover, extra caution is required for the diagnosis of hypothyroidism in older adults because signs of fatigue, weakness, constipation, dry skin, and inability to tolerate cold can be attributed to diseases other than hypothyroidism in this age group. Additionally, the side effects of multiple medications in the elderly can mask and even reproduce some of the signs and symptoms of hypothyroidism.

Another study compared the number of signs or symptoms of hypothyroidism between older (seventy-nine years of age on average) and younger patients (forty-one years on average) and concluded that the older group had just under seven signs or symptoms and the younger group had slightly more than nine. Fatigue and weakness were the most common complaints in older adults, while inability to tolerate cold, numbness in the extremities, weight gain, and abdominal cramps were less common than in the younger group. Depression is also common to hypothyroidism in older adults and might be related to loneliness more in this group than in younger adults. Also, low activity of the thyroid in older adults has been associated with impairment of several cognitive functions, including attention and concentration, language and memory, and perceptual and spatial orientation. Severe hypothyroidism can be confused with dementias. Most of the symptoms listed above usually improve with treatment and restoration of the physiological state of the thyroid.

Oxidants (reactive oxygen species, or oxygen radicals) are required for biosynthetic processes such as the synthesis of thyroid hormones. They participate in the regulation of many cellular processes, including cell death, cell differentiation, and cell migration. In a rare form of hypothyroidism, hydrogen peroxide (an oxidant) is a necessary cofactor for the enzyme that participates in the final step in the synthesis of thyroid hormones. For years researchers studying the thyroid gland have been searching for an enzyme that produces hydrogen peroxide. They have discovered that dual oxidase two (DUOX2) generates the hydrogen peroxide required for the biochemical function of thyroid peroxidase. DUOX2 was first identified in the mammalian thyroid gland but has since been found in other vertebrates, including humans, and in lower forms of life such as insects, nematodes, fungi, amoeba, alga, and plants. These enzymes clearly have a single function: to regulate the production of reactive oxygen species. They have been implicated in hypertension, immunity, hearing, and the synthesis of thyroid hormones.

The Aging Pancreas

The mammalian pancreas gland has both endocrine and exocrine functions. The primary endocrine hormones of the human pancreas are insulin and glucagon. These hormones are secreted into the pancreatic blood, delivered to the general systemic circulation, and then transported to their target tissues (such as muscle). The primary exocrine products of the pancreas gland are bicarbonate ion (HCO_3^-) and digestive enzymes (for example, pancreatic lipases). These pancreatic products are not secreted into the circulating blood. Rather, they are released into small ducts that form a main pancreatic duct that converges with the common bile duct (from the gallbladder) and then drains into the duodenum. In the small intestine, bicarbonate ions buffer gastric acids, and pancreatic lipases help digest and process dietary fats (exocrine functions).

The incidence and prevalence of type II diabetes increase with age, and the disease now affects up to 30 percent of the elderly population in the United States. It has been hypothesized that insulin resistance increases with age due to increased adipose tissue, decreased lean muscle mass, changes in dietary habits, and reduced physical activity. The underlying physiological mechanisms are still poorly understood. However, these factors alone cannot account for age-related intolerance to glucose. Many researchers have conducted studies in humans to clarify the mechanism by which glucose intolerance develops. But early investigations of the age-related increase in peripheral resistance to insulin yielded inconclusive results. For example, in one study comparing young (ages eighteen to thirty-six years) and older (ages fifty-seven to eighty-two years) men, investigators found a significant decrease in the metabolic clearance rate for glucose in the older subjects despite elevated circulating concentrations of insulin in their plasma. Such results imply that insulin sensitivity decreases with age. In another study of young (ages nineteen to thirty-six years) and older (ages forty-seven to seventy-three years) men, the metabolic clearance of plasma glucose was found to be associated with the waist-to-hip ratio but not with age. This implies that the content and distribution of abdominal fat, and not age alone, affects insulin resistance.

Studies of the effects of age on pancreatic beta cells have also yielded inconsistent results. One European study revealed a 25 percent decline in the rate of delivery of insulin from age eighteen to age eighty-five. That investigation controlled for body mass index, fasting plasma glucose, and insulin sensitivity in both men and women. Its results suggested that the functioning of beta cells declines with age. In contrast, in a study of young (ages twenty-three to twenty-five years) and older (ages sixty-four to sixty-six years) adults, defects in the function of beta cells in older subjects were observed only with preexisting impaired glucose tolerance or type II diabetes. Older subjects and younger ones with similar physiological glucose profiles also had similar insulin responses to experimental hyperglycemia. These results suggest that there is not necessarily an overall age-related decrease in the function of beta cells, and decreased function might be observed only in people with diabetes.

The incidence of diabetes increases with age, and there are multiple possible explanations for this fact. For example, it may be that the proliferative capacity of beta cells is reduced with age. There also seems to be an increased rate of cellular apoptosis of beta cells as we age. Reduced expression of activators or increased expression of inhibitors of the cell cycle are among the mechanisms that could explain these observations. Increased aggregation of islet amyloid polypeptide (amylin) is another mechanism that has attracted considerable attention. Amylin is a neuroendocrine hormone that is secreted along with insulin from pancreatic beta cells. Amylin suppresses secretion of glucagon and helps regulate glucose homeostasis in the presence of insulin. In type II diabetes, elevated secretion of insulin accompanies increased secretion of amylin. Excess amylin aggregates into amyloid plaques and leads to increased apoptosis of beta cells, causing the progression of diabetes.

At autopsy, amyloid plaques are present in more than 90 percent of people who had type II diabetes. Also at autopsy, aging leads to increased deposition of amylin in the islets of the pancreas only in people who had diabetes. Interestingly, due to an amino acid substitution that makes rodent amylin different from human amylin, rodent amyloid does not aggregate. Taking advantage of this knowledge, scientists have developed transgenic mice that express the human amylin gene. Experimentally induced overexpression of amylin results in hyperglycemia in male mice six to nine months of age without the presence of amyloid plaques. In transgenic male mice older than thirteen months, there was significant formation of amylin plaques in peripheral and perivascular areas of the pancreatic islets.

Although proliferation of beta cells occurs at a reduced pace with age, maintenance of the number of beta cells and the mass of pancreatic islets that house them is critical to the maintenance of normoglycemia (plasma concentrations of blood sugar or glucose that are within the physiological range of about 70–90). The production of insulin-producing cells in aging adults occurs predominantly through self-duplication of mature cells rather than through differentiation of their stem cell progenitors. Conversely, in younger individuals the principal mechanism—during and after development of the fetus—is the production of new beta cells by stem or precursor cells. The replication of beta cells and the mass of pancreatic islets are strictly regulated by the genetic programs in these cells, extrinsic growth factors, and circulating concentrations of hormones that respond to physiological requirements and aphysiological challenges. Disrupting the self-replicating capability of beta cells leads to a decrease in the mass of islet tissue. In turn, this reduces the production of insulin, deregulates the homeostasis of glucose, and ultimately drives hyperglycemia and diabetes. Therefore, analyzing the cellular pathways that control islet mass and understanding the mechanisms that regulate beta cell regeneration are likely to lead to new interventions for the treatment of diabetes.

It has been established that the proliferation and regeneration of beta cells is controlled through proteins of the cell cycle and their precursors. Additionally, damage to DNA and the reactive cellular responses permanently halt the beta cell cycle, leading to diabetes. Regardless of the stimuli used to foster regeneration of beta cells, they must all converge on the replicative machinery of the basic cell cycle. This cycle is a highly regulated succession of subcellular events that is responsible for cellular replication and the homeostasis of cell numbers, tissue mass, and functioning of organs and organ systems.

Since the main mechanism for generation of beta cells is self-renewal, it might be desirable to manipulate such regulation in the search for therapies. One potential starting point is the knowledge that deregulation of the cell cycle will halt proliferation of beta cells and trigger cellular aging, subsequently causing metabolic disorder and type II diabetes. To avoid this problem, scientists need to find targets that relieve the proliferative restriction placed on beta cells without driving the development of new cells and islets (leading to metastasis, or cancer). Unfortunately, many upstream regulators that influence the cell cycle and control proliferation of beta cells have not been discovered. Moreover, the effects of genomic and individual stresses such as those induced by diets high in fats, sugars, and calories, as well as the roles of DNA repair and damage, still remain unclear.

In summary, like the nervous system, the endocrine system is a communications and regulations system. It is next to impossible to think of a cell, tissue, or organ that is not affected by both systems. Moreover, like the nervous and all other human organ systems, aging takes its toll on the endocrine system. Evidence of this is seen in the age-related malfunction of any one or more of the multiple endocrine organs. Finally, like all other human organ systems, unequivocal experimental results reveal that exercising self-control in matters of diet and physical activity during the life span is still one of the best ways to ensure good endocrine health into old age. An apple a day might never have kept the doctor away, but a run—or swim or walk—a day will help keep disease away.

4

The Aging Immune System

On Friday, October 4, 2013, I had my most recent physical exam. I see my doctor for such purposes each year. I was already scheduled to have my annual flu shot at work the following Friday. After the exam, my doctor asked, "Have you had your pneumonia shot?" I told him I had never heard of such a shot. He said that as we age, our immune systems weaken, and that health agencies in the United States advise older people to get an annual pneumonia shot. I agreed, and his nurse gave me the injection. One week later I had my flu shot.

It was easy for me to see the logic of my doctor's reasoning. I am aging. And earlier in the year I had come in contact with an allergen or pathogen that caused small skin lesions on both forearms (contact dermatitis). At the time, I was seeing a dermatologist for treatment of a basal cell skin cancer in my right ear. I showed her the forearm lesions, and she didn't seem concerned but advised me to watch them for the next several weeks. That was in May or June 2013. By the end of October 2013, the lesions had disappeared from my right arm but not the left. These experiences caused me to think about the comparative health of the immune systems in the skin of my forearms and ears. They also made me wonder about the immunity of other bilaterally arranged but internal organs such as my kidneys, lungs, and cerebral hemispheres.

The standard mammalian organ systems—including the cardiovascular, respiratory, and renal systems—are well known, but some people would argue that there is no organized immune system. Still, immunity has been revealed to be one of the most complex functions of the human body. Simply defined, immunity is the physiological state of having sufficient defenses to avoid infection, disease, or other unwanted pathological invasions of the body. In short, it is the capability of the body to resist harmful pathogens. Immunity begins with the skin but also includes specialized cells at every portal in the body, such as the oral cavity, respiratory passageways, and other orifices. When the immune system malfunctions, it can not only fail to protect the body but can also attack it. Even normal, healthy aging is accompanied by impaired immune function.

Studies describing specific alterations in the aging immune system are often contradictory, and the degree of change and reproducibility of observations vary with the clinical status of the elderly and their coexisting disease. The greatest variation occurs in the most impaired elderly, including those in nursing homes. For example, there is a consistent decline in immune cells found in the lymph nodes and lymphatic circulations in the institutionalized elderly. This might be important in the reactivation of shingles or tuberculosis. Also, the elderly show diminished production of antibodies to both pneumonia and influenza vaccines. Moreover, they are often unable to avoid noxious environments that can further compromise their immune systems. Consider bedridden nursing home residents whose rooms are near the outside entrances to the buildings. Residents, staff members, and visitors who smoke are rarely more than a few feet away from these entrances during their cigarette breaks, and the smoke often reaches nearby residents. As a visitor to such facilities, I've been forced to breathe this secondhand smoke. This smoke is unhealthy for the bedridden residents and their immune systems.

The body defends itself from major seasonal diseases such as influenza, hay fever, and related allergies through its immune system. In the first few months of 2013, the former president of South Africa, Nelson Mandela, was hospitalized several times for influenza and other complications of aging. He died on December 5, 2013, at age ninety-five. The world paid tribute to this inspirational leader for several weeks after. Toward the end of 2012, when he was in his late eighties, Ed Koch, the former mayor of New York City, was hospitalized for similar conditions. He died of influenza-related complications in February 2013. Senator Frank Lautenberg of New Jersey died in June 2013 from viral influenza. At age eighty-nine, he was the oldest veteran of World War II then serving in the US Senate—in fact, he was the oldest senator. Lautenberg was given a funeral with full military honors and was buried in Arlington National Cemetery.

Influenza can lead to cardiovascular and respiratory complications, which are among the six leading causes of catastrophic disability. As the US population ages, rising rates of hospitalization are anticipated from seasonal influenza. The impact of influenza on disability and frailty in older adults is only beginning to be understood. Rates of long-term morbidity and disability following influenza in older people are predictable, and it is difficult to discuss the aging immune system without considering the impacts of influenza on it. In the event of a real flu pandemic among the elderly, the cost of hospitalization could threaten to paralyze the country's health care system and related social systems of support.

In the elderly, the flu is increasingly recognized as an illness that goes well beyond the statistics of pneumonia and influenza. In adults ages seventy years and older, peak mortality due to respiratory illness and also ischemic heart disease, cerebrovascular events, and diabetes coincides with cyclic, annual epidemics of influenza. This suggests that the flu is a major cause of excess mortality in this population during the winter months. Moreover, death rates and hospitalization during flu season are rising in spite of the widespread vaccinations implemented in the 1990s. On average, influenza resulted in 36,000 deaths annually in the United States from 1990 to 1999, almost double the annual number for the period from 1980 to 1989.

A similar rise in the rates of hospitalization for acute respiratory illnesses and cardiovascular diseases during flu season was also observed over these two time periods. The marked increase in rates of serious influenza is due, in part, to the rising prevalence of conditions of high risk, including cardiovascular diseases, in people ages sixty-five years and older. With improved health care, advances in medicine, and the aging of the baby boomers, in conjunction with the marked decline in the birth rate, the percentage of the US population ages sixty-five years and older is steadily increasing. For the elderly and the nation as a whole, vaccination programs are cost-saving even though vaccines often fail to provide adequate protection. Unfortunately, influenza continues to have devastating consequences in the elderly.

Changes in the aging immune system not only result in reduced response to vaccination and reduced protection against influenza, but they also present significant challenges to the development of new vaccines. In older adults, the goal is to provide clinical protection against the disease rather than to enhance immunity. Rising numbers of hospitalizations and rates of death due to influenza over the past two decades lead to calls for more effective flu vaccines for the elderly. A greater understanding of how age-related changes and their interactions with common chronic diseases is also needed. There have been major advances in the technology of vaccination, but the clinical and pharmaceutical development of new vaccines is dependent on the production of antibodies as an indicator of efficacy and protection.

Many of the physiological alterations in all the major organ systems with aging contribute to the development of infection. For instance, age-related changes in the skin cause delayed healing of wounds. Changes in the function and structure of the respiratory tract increase the likelihood of aspiration (taking the contents of meals, liquefied or otherwise, into the trachea versus the esophagus) and pneumonia. Alterations in gastrointestinal physiology such as decreased gastric acidity increase the likelihood of infection after the ingestion of pathogens. And the urinary tract is more vulnerable to infection with old age in both women and men, even in the absence of other diseases.

As a consequence of the aging-related changes identified above, there has been a paradigm shift in how we measure the efficacy of influenza vaccine in older people: we now understand the limitations of relying solely on circulating concentrations of antibodies for this measurement. In the elderly, adequate levels of antibodies might not provide immunity because antibodies fail to bind viruses and to prevent infection of cells. One challenge to the development of new vaccines is taking into consideration the aging immune system in a growing fraction of the population. Another is using concentrations of antibodies in the plasma as a sole predictor of the efficacy of vaccines. This might fail to detect other markers of immunity that enhance protection in older people. For example, as we age, we lose body mass in general (that is, the losses are not limited to muscle). The distribution of body water can change with age, and a related potential change is a decrease in circulating plasma volume. An age-related decrease in plasma volume could increase the concentration of a desirable drug in the circulation, thereby making it more effective in supplementing immunity or fighting infection.

The Innate Immune System

Immunity involves specific and nonspecific elements. The nonspecific component (innate immunity) acts either as a barrier, such as the skin, or as an eliminator of a wide range of pathogens. The specific component adapts to each new disease or to a single pathogen (adaptive immunity). Innate immunity is the natural resistance with which a person is born. It is the dominant system of defense in most organisms playing host to an invading pathogen. In order for airborne pathogens to enter the body, they must first pass through epithelial/endothelial layers of cells, the primary physical barriers that help define our skin and mucous membranes. Secondary molecular and physiological barriers (the humoral component) include chemical secretions such as cytokines (which act as messengers to other parts of the body) and antimicrobials, fever and hyperthermia that can detoxify and impair foreign invaders, and phagocytosis that is associated with general inflammatory responses. Humoral components can also include vasodilators that increase blood flow and hasten the delivery of antibodies to a site of infection, or the removal of pathogens from the same site. Such agents include histamine, bradykinin, and a host of others.

Phagocytes are white blood cells that can ingest and detoxify pathogens and the harmful substances they release. Phagocytes also produce receptors at their cell surfaces that can respond to common molecular patterns found on the surfaces of invading pathogens. Through these physical, molecular, and physiological mechanisms, innate immunity prevents the entry, colonization, and spread of pathogens in humans. Related physical barriers protect lower forms of animal life as well as plants from diseases and infection. The waxy film on leaves; the exoskeleton of insects; the peels of bananas and oranges and the skin of onions; and the shells and membranes of edible eggs are only a few examples of the first line of defense against invasion by pathogens.

For better or worse, however, humans, other animals, and plants cannot be completely sealed off from their environments. Therefore, other immune defenses act to protect ports of entry such as the mouth and respiratory tract, the urogenital orifices, and the eyes and ears. In the pulmonary system, coughing and sneezing mechanically eject pathogens and other irritants from the respiratory tract. Still other inhaled or aspirated agents get embedded in mucosal secretions. These are moved in an alveolar-to-oral direction by ciliated epithelia (respiratory escalators). Ciliated epithelia are cells whose luminal borders have hairlike projections that interact with the air flowing past them. Additionally, the flushing action of tears and urine mechanically expels some pathogens.

The body's cells and tissues secrete antimicrobial products and other chemical barriers such as enzymes in saliva, tears, and breast milk. Additionally, following the onset of the monthly menstrual cycle, vaginal secretions serve as chemical barriers (the secretions become slightly acidic), while semen contains related enzymes and zinc to kill pathogens. In the stomach, gastric or hydrochloric acid and proteases (enzymes that break down proteins) serve as lethal chemical defenses against ingested pathogens. In the urogenital and gastrointestinal tracts, residential fauna and flora also serve as biological barriers. These microbial animal and plant species compete with pathogenic bacteria for food and space and can change physiological conditions in the environment (for example, by altering pH). Such beneficial changes reduce the probability that pathogens will reach sufficient numbers to cause illness.

Since most antibiotics target bacteria generically and do not kill fungi, oral antibiotics can lead to fungal overgrowth and can cause illnesses such as vaginal yeast infections. There is growing evidence that replenishing depleted intestinal flora helps restore gastrointestinal balance (homeostasis) in infected children. It can also be useful for adults suffering from bacterial gastroenteritis, inflammatory bowel syndrome, urinary tract infections, and post-surgical infections. Such gastrointestinal balance can be achieved in many cases simply by eating probiotic yogurt, which contains pure cultures of lactobacilli in an unpasteurized state.

The innate immune system does not confer long-lasting immunity, and its response is usually triggered when cellular receptors recognize patterns that are present in broad groups of microorganisms (such as specific proteins on various pathogens). It is also activated when damaged or injured cells release distress signals, such as during inflammation. Inflammation is one of the first responses of the immune system to infection and tissue injury. Latin terminology for the symptoms of inflammation includes the words *calor* (heat, or calories), *dolor* (pain), *rubor* (redness), and *tumor* (swelling, or cancer). Individually and collectively, these symptoms reflect changes in the physiological homeostasis of the circulatory and immune systems in the infected or injured tissues. The reader might also recognize the above symptoms as evidence of increased blood flow to the site of injury, which can lead to redness and pain—that is, increased blood flow can cause tissue edema or swelling and compression of sensory nerves.

Inflammation and tissue swelling (edema) are caused primarily by an imbalance of vascular and tissue forces (called Starling forces) that help regulate blood volume and blood flow in the microcirculation of the injured tissues. The interested reader can learn more about Starling forces in another book I wrote, *Our Marvelous Bodies* (Rutgers University Press, 2008). Damaged tissues release pro-inflammatory molecules, among many other chemicals. These molecules have unusual names such as eiconsanoids and leukotrienes. Eicosanoids are synthesized from fat-like molecules called prostaglandins. They can produce fever and cause vasodilation and vasoconstriction. Cytokines such as leukotrienes attract white blood cells and platelets to the site of injury. Platelets are also called thrombocytes because they cause thrombosis (clotting). Other common cytokines include interleukins, which are responsible for cell-to-cell communication; chemotaxins, or chemicals that promote movement of cells and molecules to the site of damage or infection; and interferons, which have antiviral effects such as shutting down protein synthesis in the host cell. Growth factors and cytotoxic factors might also be released during tissue injury.

Among the physiological requirements of the injured tissues is the need to regulate the ratio of oxygen supply to oxygen demand. The homeostasis of oxygen supply and demand is a blood flow and vascular problem. It is most satisfactorily addressed by the production and release of controlling vasodilator and vasoconstrictor substances whose job is to help restore balance among flow, pressure, and resistance. Correspondingly, cytokines and other chemicals recruit immune cells to the site of infection. Cytokines act jointly with physiological forces to help restore oxygen balance and to promote healing after pathogens have been removed.

The complement system, a subset of the general immune system, is a cascade of internal biochemicals that attacks the surfaces of foreign cells. The complement system contains multiple proteins and is named for its ability to aid the killing of pathogens by antibodies. It is the major tissue component of the innate immune response. Many species—including plants, fish, and some invertebrates—have complement systems. In humans, this subsystem is activated by the binding of complement proteins either to antibodies that have already attached themselves to pathogens or to carbohydrates and other molecules on the surfaces of pathogens. Peptides are then produced that attract immune cells; increase microvascular permeability to them; and coat the surface of pathogens, thus marking them for destruction. Deposition of complement proteins can also kill cells directly by disrupting their plasma membranes. The binding of complement proteins to a pathogen triggers a rapid killing response: the activation of proteases uses positive feedback to amplify the initial signal. The signal can be transmitted to the central nervous system, bone marrow, the liver, and/or other organs involved in synthesizing or releasing complement. It is thought that the complement system plays a role in many diseases with an immune component, including arthritis, asthma, inflammatory bowel syndrome, lupus, and multiple sclerosis.

Cellular Barriers and the Immune System

Leukocytes (white blood cells) act like independent single-cell organisms and constitute the second arm of the innate immune system. These cells include macrophages and neutrophils (both of which are phagocytes), mast cells, dendritic cells, and natural killer cells. Macrophages and neutrophils are leukocytes that circulate in the bloodstream and then take up residency in soft tissues and bone. Mast cells are ubiquitous and commonly release histamine and other edema-causing agents during inflammation and allergic responses. Dendritic cells act like macrophages and neutrophils and are not to be confused with dendritic cells of the central and peripheral nervous systems. And natural killer cells are leukocytes that attack and destroy tumor cells or cells that have been infected by viruses. They got their name because they do not require activation to destroy cells.

Phagocytes identify and eliminate pathogens by engulfing and killing them intracellularly (phagocytosis). Phagocytosis is an important feature of cellular immunity in people of all ages, and it is one of the oldest forms of defense in vertebrates and invertebrates. Phagocytes generally patrol the body searching for pathogens (much like the game of Pac-Man) but can be attracted to specific locations by cytokines. Once a pathogen has been detected by a phagocyte, it engulfs the pathogen, trapping it inside an intracellular vesicle called the phagosome. Inside the vesicle, pathogens are killed by the activity of digestive enzymes or by the release of toxic free radicals.

Among white blood cells, neutrophils are the most abundant phagocytes in people of all ages. They represent as much as 60 percent of the total leukocyte pool. During the acute phase of infection, neutrophils migrate to the site of injury in a process called chemotaxis. Chemotaxis means that the infected cells release cytokines and other neurohumors that are recognized by the traveling white blood cells (that is, the two chemicals attract each other). Stationary white blood cells (macrophages), on the other hand, take up residency in soft tissue and bone after a brief period in the circulation. They produce and release enzymes, complement proteins, and regulatory factors. Macrophages act as scavengers that rid the body of worn-out cells and other debris. Not surprisingly, age diminishes both the numbers and activity of neutrophils and macrophages. Both become less effective in removing aged cells and debris as one gets older. For example, of the 36,000 people who die from influenza in the United States in an average year, about 90 percent are sixty-five years of age and older. Older individuals also have a higher incidence of bacterial infections in the lungs, urinary tract, skin, and other soft tissues. Infections in the elderly are also more severe and more likely to result in fatalities than those in younger people. A growing body of evidence suggests that this increased incidence of infections results from defects in the ability of epithelial cells, macrophages, and neutrophils to function as effective immune barriers in the elderly.

Another type of immune cell that is affected by age is the mast cell. On the basis of their unique staining characteristics and large granules, mast cells were among the first immune cells to be described. Two types of mast cell are known: those produced in connective tissue and mucosal mast cells. Mast cells contain histamine and anticoagulants like heparin. They release histamine on binding to immunoglobulins. Mast cells and basophils (white blood cells that pick up alkaline stains) are thought to originate in the bone marrow. Basophils are mature when they leave the bone marrow, whereas mast cells circulate in an immature state. The tissue site that an immature mast cell settles in probably determines its precise mature characteristics and the influences of aging on these. Mast cells are found surrounding blood vessels and nerves and are especially prominent near the boundaries between the outside world and the inside of the body, such as the skin and mucosa of the lungs, digestive tract, mouth, eyes, and nose. Mast cells play a key role in the inflammatory process. When activated, they rapidly release secretory granules into the interstitium. Mast cells can be stimulated to release their granules by direct chemical or physical injury, by cross-talk among immunoglobulins, or by activated complement proteins. Mast cells are coated with immunoglobulin E, which is responsive to a specific class of antigens.

Anyone who has suffered from seasonal allergies has experienced mast cells in action. If your eyes itch, you probably rub them for relief. After rubbing, you might notice them reddening. Among other things, the reddening is due to release of histamine, the mechanical agitation of the rubbing and the accompanying vasodilation, and increased permeability of the small blood vessels of the eyes. Histamine and related chemicals are also responsible for your stuffed-up nostrils. In the nostrils, the histamine-mediated increase in permeability causes mucosal edema and inflammation. The congested mucosa of the nasal passageways makes it difficult to breathe and talk. Moreover, if the airborne allergens in hay fever season contact your skin, they can cause rashes that are particularly noticeable in the sweating skin folds (such as in the neck, elbow joint, wrist, and other exposed skin joints). These rashes are also caused by release of histamine and related chemicals, such as bradykinin.

Dendritic cells are phagocytes that are in contact with the external environment. They serve as links between the tissues and the innate and adaptive immune systems. Dendritic cells are also found at ports of entry for pathogens and other foreign matter. This means they reside in the skin and epithelial mucosal membranes lining the nasal passages, the respiratory bronchioles and other airways, the stomach, intestinal tract, and urogenital orifices and channels. Like mast cells, they are also present in the eyes and ears. Dendritic cells are named for their resemblance to neuronal dendrites but are not functional components of the nervous system. For example, they do not generate action potentials, release neurotransmitters, or synthesize insulating material such as myelin sheaths.

Adaptive and Cellular Immunity

The adaptive immune system complements the innate immune system as well as creating immunological memory, in which each pathogen is remembered by a signature antigen. The adaptive immune response is antigen-specific and requires the recognition of specific foreign antigens. Antigen specificity is tailored to specific pathogens, and the ability to mount these tailored immune responses is maintained by memory cells. Should a pathogen infect the body more than once, for example, specific memory cells quickly eliminate it when it returns. Throughout the lifetime of an animal or human, such memory cells retain the ability to identify specific pathogens and can mount strong and repetitive responses each time the pathogen is detected.

Immunological memory comes in the form of either passive, short-term memory or active, long-term memory. The cells of the adaptive immune system are lymphocytes called B and T cells, which are derived from the bone marrow. B cells are involved in humoral immune responses, whereas T cells are involved in cell-mediated immune responses. (Humoral means functioning in the circulation and other body fluids.) Both B and T cells carry receptor molecules that recognize specific targets. T cells recognize a foreign pathogen after its antigens have been presented to the body. B cells (also referred to as plasma cells because they produce antibodies) identify pathogens when the cells' antibodies bind to specific foreign antigens. The subsequent antigen-antibody complex is transferred into the B cell and processed by the breakdown of proteins into smaller peptides. Matching helper T cells release lymphokines to activate the B cell, which divides, creating daughter cells. The daughter cells of multiple activated B cells then secrete millions of copies of antibodies that recognize corresponding antigens. Such antibodies circulate in blood plasma and lymph, bind to pathogens expressing the antigen, and mark them for destruction.

A baby's immune system is not fully developed until he or she is about six months old. Several layers of passive protection are provided by mothers. First, during pregnancy, immunoglobulin G (IgG) is transported from maternal to fetal blood directly across the placental membrane barrier. IgG antibodies are the smallest antibodies, but they make up 75 percent of all antibodies in the body. They are present in all body fluids and are considered to be the most important antibodies in the fight against bacterial and viral infections. These antibodies help protect the fetus from developing an infection inside the womb. Immediately after birth, the newborn has high levels of the mother's antibodies in the bloodstream.

Babies who are breastfed continue to receive antibodies via breast milk, the second layer of passive protection. Breast milk contains all five types of antibodies: immunoglobulins A, D, E, G, and M. These antibodies are delivered to the baby's gut and protect the infant until he or she can synthesize antibodies independently. (Similarly, passive immunity can be transferred artificially from a donor to a recipient using antibody-rich plasma.) During the next several months the antibodies passed from the mother to the infant steadily decrease. When healthy babies are about two to three months old, their immune system will start producing its own antibodies. During this time the baby will experience the body's natural low point of antibodies in the bloodstream. This is because the maternal antibodies have decreased, and infants who are making antibodies for the first time do so at a much slower rate than adults. Once healthy babies reach about six months of age, they are producing antibodies at normal adult rates.

An immune response begins with initial exposure to a pathogen (or initial vaccination) and leads to the formation and maintenance of active immunological memory. Long-term active memory or immunity is acquired through activation of the B and T cells mentioned above. Active memory can also be achieved artificially through vaccination. The principle behind vaccination is to introduce a foreign antigen from a less virulent pathogen—either from dead or living pathogen—that stimulates the development of active immunity without causing the disease associated with the pathogen. This deliberate induction of an antigen-antibody response is successful because it exploits the natural specificity and inducibility of the immune system.

With infectious disease being one of the leading causes of death in the human population, vaccinations represent effective manipulations of the immune system. Most viral vaccines are based on live attenuated viruses, while many bacterial vaccines are derived from noncellular components of bacteria. Since many antigens derived from noncellular vaccines do not strongly induce the adaptive response, most bacterial vaccines are provided with additional adjuvants that activate the antigen-presenting cells of the innate immune system. In this regard, the development of new drugs will always be challenged as unknown pathogens continue to be identified and activities of existing toxins unfold. One such example is the bacterium *Escherichia coli*. It was once thought to be limited to communicable diseases. However, as research in the past half-century has shown *E. coli* plays major roles in burn trauma, metabolic shock, and wound healing, for example.

Experiments using the common laboratory mouse have helped advance knowledge of the aging immune system. However, it is important to emphasize that there are fundamental and significant differences between mice and humans in the species' basic immunology. For example, mice have immunoproteins that are a natural component of the cellular or tissue milieu. But immunoproteins in humans must be induced—that is, they are not a standard option in that milieu. Other differences between the mouse and human immune systems include the unique primate genes that encode for immunoglobulin-like receptors in natural killer cells and whether selected proteins in the T cells serve to activate (in mice) or inhibit (in humans). Perhaps the best example of species-specific differences is a gene-protein complex called cluster of differentiation (CD) 28, which is expressed on T cells throughout the life of mice but is irreversibly lost with aging in humans. CD28 is a protein structure that one T cell needs to be recognized by other cells. These and other differences underscore the need for caution when trying to translate laboratory observations in mice to humans.

Moreover, the experimental settings are consistently different between mice and men as well. Experiments in mice are generally performed in a regulated, sanitized, and highly controlled laboratory environment. Naturally, experimental environments for humans are less sanitized and less controlled. For many years my office and experimental and teaching laboratories have been in the same building, and adjacent to the university's animal care facilities, which are approved by the Association for Assessment and Accreditation of Laboratory Animal Care. Oh, what a difference! My trashcans are emptied semiregularly, but my multiple requests to have the floors in my space swept, mopped, and vacuumed have been met with great resistance from housekeeping staff members and supervisors. Conversely, the animals I use have their housing conditions maintained on a daily basis by a staff of veterinarians and certified laboratory animal care technicians. For example, the bedding of rodents is replaced regularly, and their cages or containers are washed and sanitized daily. I rarely if ever enter our vivarium without seeing multiple laboratory animal care technicians regularly working to maintain the animals' space.

Aging B and T Cells

Prior to the mid-twentieth century, the thymus was not thought to be involved in immunity in mice in the same way it is in humans. In the 1950s investigators began removing the thymus from newborn mice. The earlier the glands were removed, the more impaired the immune function seemed to be. The most critical period for removing the glands was before one week of life. When the glands were removed later—that is,when the mouse's lymphatic system and the immune mechanisms had partially developed—only negligible effects were observed. These early experiments indicate that: (1) removal of the thymus is associated with reduced numbers of lymphocytes; (2) the earlier in life the thymus is removed, the greater the deficiency of lymphocytes in other organs; and (3) although removing the thymus in adult mice diminishes the production of lymphocytes, it does not stop it—which is not the case in newborns.

Like all other organs and tissues of the mammalian body, the thymus is subject to the effects of aging, and humans and mice show some similarities in immune function with age. For example, T cells are found in both mice and humans. T cells can be distinguished from other lymphocytes such as B cells and natural killer cells by the presence of a Toll-like receptor on their cell surfaces. The activity of T cells is used as a biomarker to estimate aging in the immune system, since nearly all of the cells' functions are reduced by aging. As we age, T cells produce fewer cytokines, the diversity of cytokines produced decreases, their physiological homeostasis is modified, and their proliferation is impaired. Individually and collectively, the intracellular signal transduction capability of T cells is less regulated with age, and T cells become less cytotoxic. Although not all functions of the Toll-like receptors are adversely affected by age, impaired signaling of particular Toll-like receptors impedes the synthesis and degradation of selected proteins. Age-related dysfunction of the turnover of Toll-like receptors predicts broader disruption of protein status quo, as cells naturally undergo aging or experience acute conditions of pathophysiology.

Age-related functional alterations among T cells are highlighted by deficits in signaling, changes in co-stimulatory signals, altered production of cytokines, and increased numbers of inhibitory receptors. For example, with persistent viral infections there is the natural need to produce virus-specific T cells throughout life. However, due to the wear and tear of aging, many antigen-specific T cells have pronounced functional defects—which makes it impossible for them to provide protection against viral reinfection or reactivation.

There is also an apparent difference in the pattern of some viral infections between the elderly in Europe and the United States. For example, Europeans become infected with large viruses more slowly with age, but testing positive for that virus in elderly Europeans has been associated with poor health outcomes. In contrast, there is more widespread positive testing for large viruses in the US population due to exposure at an earlier age. Other studies report increased expression of natural killer receptors on T cells in elderly people in the United States. An interesting topic for future research would be to examine the contribution made by natural killer–like T cells to the protective immunity of the aged on different continents, particularly in centenarians and supercentenarians who might have unusual immune physiology.

Another class of lymphocytes is the B cell. B cells make up the humoral branch of the adaptive immune system. The principal functions of B cells are to make antibodies against antigens, perform the role of antigen-presenting cells, and become memory B cells after initial activation by antigens. B cells can be distinguished from other lymphocytes, such as T cells and natural killer cells, by the presence of a protein on the outer surface of the cell membrane known as a B cell receptor. This specialized protein allows B cells to bind to specific antigens and allergens.

During an immune response, B cells can switch the expression of surface antibodies from immunoglobulin M to immunoglobulins A, E, and G. These switches require modifications of the S regions of the immunoglobulins, molecular recognition, cleavage of the target DNA by selective enzymes, and repair and recombination of the cleaved ends of the antibody—thus, they are called class switch recombinations. The process is important for the humoral immune response because it generates antibodies of the same specificity but with different functions. Although rare, patients who cannot switch their immunoglobulin class have been described by researchers. Such patients have genetic defects on T cells that are required to trigger B cells. They are susceptible to bacterial and enteroviral infections, as well as to other infections. They not only possess a defect in class switch recombination that is characterized by the lack of production of immunoglobulins A, E, and G, but their antibodies are also defective in the ability to develop mature affinity characteristics. These patients frequently have upper and lower respiratory tract infections, otitis, diarrhea, oral ulcers, and autoimmunity. They fail to respond to vaccination, and their condition worsens with age.

There is an increasing trend for functionally exhausted, switched-memory B cells to accumulate with age. It appears that this pool of aged naive B cells—cells that have not been exposed to antigens—is markedly increased among centenarians, which raises the question of whether there is an undiscovered role for naive B cells that could be beneficial in extreme old age. For example, what if a pool of aged naive B cells from an older experimental animal could be transplanted into a young animal? Would the younger recipient then mature with a healthier immune system that could be passed on to its offspring? Answers to questions like this are still awaiting experimentation. With a life span of only a few days, many B cells die without ever encountering their activating antigens and becoming activated when their receptors bind to the antigens. Once naive B cells have been exposed to antigens, they become either memory B cells or plasma cells that release antibodies specific to the antigen that originally caused their maturation. Investigators have reported that the proportion of naive B cells increases with age. This phenomenon is not due to the accelerated formation of new B cells but to alterations in the memory-switching machinery of immunoglobulins.

The functioning of B cells in aging can suffer from lack of help from T cells, but changes intrinsic to B cells also occur. This can have a significant impact on the production and function of antibodies. Intrinsic changes refer to functions of B cells that do not require external stimuli. Aging-related intrinsic changes include decreases in nuclear DNA or RNA, reduced production of IgG, and diminished response to stimulation by the flu virus. Objectives of research in this area include identifying biomarkers of the human B cell and correlating these with physiological immune responses such as those that occur after influenza vaccination. The number of immature precursors to human B cells in the bone marrow has been shown to decline modestly or to remain relatively constant with age. Conversely, the number of mature human B cells significantly decreases with age. This is one reason why older people get sick more often and tend to recover more slowly and less effectively.

As an example, one group of investigators analyzed the composition of the pool of peripheral B cells in people eighteen to eighty-six years of age. The investigators found that the number of cells that produce immunoglobulin A or G decreases with age. Similar research revealed that both the percentages and actual numbers of total CD19-bearing B cells also decrease with age. The percentage of naive B cells increases with age, but the actual numbers were found to be similar in young and older subjects.

Memory B cells are a central component of humoral immunity. In contrast to plasma cells, which have only short lives in the systemic circulation, memory B cells last for years or even decades. Investigators in one laboratory demonstrated that memory B cells specific to smallpox vaccine lasted for more than fifty years in immunized individuals. These cells were still able to mount a robust antibody response upon revaccination. Such results show that immunological memory to smallpox vaccination is long-lived and can still contribute to protection against disease many years later. Moreover, in the human tonsil, naive B cells have been shown to increase through young adulthood but then wane with age. This means the capacity to fight infections such as tonsillitis improves as we pass from childhood to young adulthood but might be impaired thereafter. A reduction in IgM-producing cells depletes specific antibodies in elderly people who have been vaccinated against pneumonia.

Finally, in the lymph nodes, mature B lymphocytes proliferate, differentiate, mutate, and then switch antibodies during a normal immune response to an infection. Germinal centers in lymph nodes are an important part of the B-cell humoral immune system. The dynamic development of such germ centers and the B lymphocytes they produce occurs following activation of B cells by T-dependent antigen. Such functional B lymphocytes have to interact with helper T cells to complete their differentiation. This involves a change from manufacturing antibodies of one type to producing those of another type—for example, from immunoglobulin M to G. Their interaction with T cells is believed to prevent the generation of autoimmune antibodies. The significant age-dependent decrease in switch memory B cells and the corresponding increase in the percentage of naive and IgM-producing memory B cells suggest an intrinsic defect in the ability of aging B cells to survive and therefore to combat infection.

In addition to the above effects of aging on B and T cells, there is mounting evidence of age-related changes in the function of dendritic cells, another immune cell line. There is considerable diversity of structure and appearances in human dendritic cells, some of which have no obvious counterparts in the mouse. Dendritic cells are present in tissues that are in contact with the external environment, such as the skin and the mucosal epithelial linings of the mouth and nose; the bronchial tree and lungs; and the esophagus, stomach, and intestines. Contact with an antigen activates dendritic cells, and they migrate to the lymph nodes where they collaborate with T and B cells to help initiate an adaptive immune response. Among other immune functions, dendritic cells serve as bridges between innate and adaptive immunity. The main functions of dendritic cells, however, are to recognize and process antigens and then present them to other cells of the immune system.

Immature dendritic cells constantly sample the surrounding environment for viruses and bacteria. They can even phagocytize small quantities of membrane from themselves (autophagocytosis) in a process called nibbling. Simultaneously, they up-regulate cell-surface receptors that activate T cells. Dendritic cells also up-regulate chemotactic receptors that attract the cells to the systemic circulation, to the spleen, or through the lymphatic circulation to lymph nodes. In these locations, immature dendritic cells present helper T cells, killer T cells, and B cells with antigens collected from the pathogens that the dendritic cells attack. Only B lymphocytes, dendritic cells, and macrophages are able to activate resting helper T cells. However, macrophages and B cells can activate only memory T cells, whereas dendritic cells can activate both memory and naive T cells. Dendritic cells are the most potent of all the antigen-presenting cells. They are also important in launching humoral immunity due, in part, to their capacity to present unprocessed antigens to B cells.

Any alterations in the functions of dendritic cells with age compromise both immunity and tolerance by affecting their capacities to phagocytose antigens, migrate to sites of infection, and secrete. The aging of dendritic cells is associated with progressive autoimmunity, immunodeficiency, and inflammation resulting in increased susceptibility to infections and impaired responses to vaccinations. This is, in part, due to a decrease in the protective immune responses of dendritic cells and to an increase in reactivity to pathogens in older individuals. Also, age-related deficiencies in immune tolerance—coupled with progressive loss of tissue integrity and memory responsiveness—place the elderly at increased risk of succumbing to disease and infections. Understanding the types and lineages of different subsets of dendritic cells is a fundamental undertaking in the development of cell-based immunotherapy.

Aging Natural Killer Cells

Natural killer cells are a type of cytotoxic lymphocyte that is critical to the innate immune system. They provide rapid responses to virally infected cells and can respond to the formation of tumors in as few as three to four days after infection. Natural killer cells are large granular lymphocytes. They are important in responses to viruses and tumors. They constitute yet another kind of cell differentiated from the common lymphoid progenitor that creates B and T lymphocytes. Natural killer cells are known to differentiate and mature in the bone marrow, lymph node, spleen, tonsils, and thymus, after which they enter the general systemic circulation. Natural killer cells are unique, however, because they have the ability to recognize stressed cells in the absence of antibodies and major histocompatibility complex. This quality is what allows them to make an accelerated immune response. Natural killer cells are another important population of cytotoxic

cells linking innate and adaptive immunities. They can kill directly without any need for previous sensitization (for example, immunization with
attenuated pathogens), binding of antibodies, or presentation of peptides.
Still, their fast and efficient ability to kill is strictly regulated. The natural
killer cell makes the decision to kill by measuring the balance between
signals received by its inhibitory and activating receptors expressed at
its surface (inhibition is dominant).

Declining numbers of natural killer cells or reductions in their functions in aging are associated with death in the elderly. In healthy elderly
people this is true even if the lethal abilities of these cells decrease.
Administration of synthetic molecules such as interleukin-2 can induce
the proliferation of natural killer cells in healthy young people, but in the
elderly the response varies from a modest decrease to no proliferation.
Interleukin-2 also modifies the secretion of cytokines by natural killer
cells. Compared to young people's cells, cells from the elderly produce less
interferon-gamma when stimulated with interleukin-2. The cytokine
interleukin-15 is another highly lethal mediator released by natural killer
cells. It might be that decreased interleukin-15 during aging constitutes a
common mechanism for muscle wasting, obesity, and immune aging.
Physiological interleukin-15 levels are rate limiting for natural killer cells.
This implies that any source of interleukin-15 will boost their cell numbers
and functions.

Skeletal muscle contributes significantly to the physiological homeostasis of natural killer cells. This implies that aging-related wasting of
muscle results in the loss of interleukin-15 and its corresponding receptors, thereby impairing the homeostasis of natural killer cells. Moreover,
when wasting of muscle is combined with elevated production of inflammatory cytokines by adipose tissue, some of which impede the function of
natural killer cells, the predicted outcome is a reduction in the numbers
and survivability of natural killer cells. This hypothesis has been tested
and validated in elderly female subjects with high body mass indexes. In
addition, chronic diseases of the heart, kidneys, and lungs are all characterized by wasting of muscle and low numbers of natural killer cells. Therefore, mechanisms that preserve the numbers and functions of natural
killer cells might promote healthy aging. Such mechanisms include sustained regular exercise, regardless of one's age. In this regard it is almost

beyond question that a lifetime of physical activity will promote a healthy immune system.

Obesity, loss of muscle mass, and low numbers of natural killer cells all predict mortality in the elderly. This suggests that these characteristics of aging might combine to promote diseases including infection and cancer. One inevitable consequence of aging in humans and other mammals (such as our pets) is sarcopenia. Some loss of muscle is due to physical inactivity, but even professionally trained athletes lose muscle mass and strength with age. Although regularly performed physical activity can delay the onset and reduce the rate of muscle deterioration, the efficacy of interventions to build muscle and to induce metabolic improvements is less efficient in the elderly than in the young. Frailty, a powerful predictor of mortality, is a clinically defined condition that includes loss of muscle mass and some of its consequences.

An increase in adipose tissue is also common with aging. Obesity and adiposity are alarming health concerns for all ages. Visceral fat is of the greatest health concern because it is associated with cancer, cardiovascular disease, dementia, insulin resistance or type II diabetes, and overall mortality. Unfortunately, the combination of obesity and loss of muscle (so-called sarcopenic obesity) carries high health risks. Although obesity can be associated with normal, decreased, or even increased muscle mass, measurements of muscle weight and the size of muscle fibers can be misleading in aging people because muscle becomes infiltrated with fat. Subcutaneous fat is part of that problem. This is fat found between the skin and underlying skeletal muscle, particularly in the abdomen and thorax. Furthermore, obesity diminishes or prevents gain of muscle in response to conditioning such as lifting weights.

Immunodeficiency and Age

Common variable immunodeficiency (AIDS-like diseases) is a heterogeneous disease characterized by impaired responses to antibodies, impaired production of immunoglobulins, recurrent infections, inflammation, and other autoimmune and malignancy-related conditions. The disease leads to repetitive infections of the respiratory, gastrointestinal, and other major organ systems. Despite private and public focus on AIDS in the past several decades, common variable immunodeficiency is the most frequent, clinically important primary immunodeficiency in humans. In the United States it has a prevalence of approximately 1 in 30,000. Until recently it had not been noticed that women suffering from this condition have significantly more switched memory B cells than men with the condition. Such women also have higher baseline concentrations of immunoglobulins A and M in their plasma than similarly affected men. These observations help explain why women with immunodeficiency-related diseases are diagnosed about a decade later in life than men, and why they outlive their male counterparts. Such infected women seem to age more successfully than men. The full details for this difference in gender are still unclear. However, circulating concentrations of IgM, a measure of B cell function, have been known for decades to be linked to the genetics and physiology of the female X chromosome.

Several women with more than one X chromosome have been examined, and a number of their genes were shown to either permit or prevent the development of B cells. Other studies have shown that the absolute numbers of B cells expressing adhesion molecules decrease in affected subjects as they age. This suggests that the ability of B cells to adhere to the inside lining of blood vessels might be impaired, and that physiological processes such as the homeostasis of clotting and hemostasis could be disrupted. On a related note, the number of B cells expressing CD38 and CD21 (compounds that help identify B cells) in the tonsils are reduced in general by age. This suggests an impairment in the first line of defense against bacterial antigens in all the elderly, not only those suffering from autoimmune diseases.

Another example of aging and immunodeficiency is the swine flu virus. The currently circulating strain of that virus mainly affects people younger than sixty years of age. This suggests that memory B cells are present in those over age sixty, and that these help control or prevent the infection. First described in April 2009, the swine flu virus appeared to be a new strain of H1N1. It resulted when an existing mixture of bird, swine, and human flu viruses combined with a Eurasian pig flu virus. Unlike most strains of influenza, H1N1 does not infect adults over age sixty disproportionately. In older individuals, at least one contributing factor is a defect in the production of antibodies (by B cells). Similarly, the production of antibodies in humans immunized against tetanus toxin, encephalitis viruses, salmonella, or pneumococcus uniformly decreases with age.

The increased frequency of infections and malignancies in elderly people not only reveals an age-associated decline of the immune system, but is also thought of by some as a condition of chronic inflammation (inflammaging). This notion is supported by the observation that elderly people have increased circulating plasma concentrations of inflammatory cytokines such as interleukin-6 and tumor necrosis factor-alpha (biomarkers of inflammation and tissue injury). The condition is combatable with anti-inflammatory steroids and other medications. However, inflammatory cytokines predict the risk of mortality independent of other risk factors. Clinical data reveal that elderly people have an increased incidence of specific chronic inflammatory diseases including chronic obstructive pulmonary disease. In addition, atherosclerosis and type II diabetes are now considered chronic inflammatory conditions that are associated with an imbalance between pro-inflammatory and anti-inflammatory cytokines.

Physical Activity and Length of
Telomeres in Aging-Related Immunity

Various approaches have been proposed to combat weakened immune defenses during aging, one of which is regular physical activity. We have all heard that a lifetime of learning is good for us. I imagine that most reasonable people agree with this. But how often do we read or hear that a lifetime of physical activity is also good for us? I believe that sustained physical activity is at least as important as sustained learning. I also believe that in time sustained physical activity will be shown to be good for healthy aging.

It is well known that middle-aged and elderly people who habitually participate in moderately intense exercise are less likely than their sedentary counterparts to develop infections. It is not known, however, if regular exercise acts only in a preventive manner to delay immunological aging, or if it can restore immunity in previously sedentary individuals. Still, it is now generally accepted that purposeful, regular physical activity is associated with a longer life span and lower risk of disease in the elderly. Should we be surprised? Exercise physiologists including my good friends

Bob Wolfe, Ed Zambraski, and Will Winder have led the charge in telling the world that regular physical activity is good for our health (their mantra for nearly five decades). More recently physicians, dieticians, nutritionists, entertainers, and others have joined the chorus.

The effects of acute exercise on immunity have been reasonably well studied in the aging, but studies examining the efficacy of chronic physical activity are lacking. The sparse data that do exist come from cross-sectional comparisons between active and inactive subjects or from randomized, controlled trials of physical activity in previously sedentary volunteers. Among the most popular measures of immune function in response to long-term physical activity are changes in numbers and appearances of T cells, in vitro proliferation of T cells to mitogens, altered titers of antibodies in response to vaccination, changes in circulating antibodies in the plasma, and the effectiveness of natural killer cells. Longitudinal experiments lasting a few months to a year or more have incorporated either active exercises (for example, running) or static ones (for example, resistance training such as weight lifting) or a combination of the two. Investigators have examined healthy middle-aged adults as well as frail, elderly residents of nursing homes and have found overall improvement with physical activity.

Pam, a colleague and younger friend of mine, has suffered from rheumatoid arthritis since her late teens. She has used multiple medications, including antibiotics, anti-inflammatories, and aspirin. On one occasion after I hadn't seen her for several weeks, I shook Pam's hand. I gripped too firmly and she grimaced. Her pained "ouch" made me feel awful. I could not apologize quickly enough. About a year before this writing, Pam began engaging in an intense exercise regimen (cycling scores of miles per week, spinning in the gym, and so forth) and was trying to improve her diet. She told me how great these activities made her feel, and how pleased she was to be able once again to twist the cap off her own bottled water, something her husband had previously had to do for her. I could hear, see, and otherwise sense her improvements. When she asked her rheumatologist to explain how the improvements had come about, the response was "I don't know."

The elderly population is at an unprecedented risk of infectious diseases and malignancy due to an apparent and inevitable age-related decline in immunity. Risk of immunity can be characterized by a profile of biomarkers that has been used to predict morbidity and mortality in older adults. During the late 1990s, a longitudinal study in a Swedish population over eighty-five years of age categorized an array of immunological parameters that could be used to predict mortality over periods of two, four, and six years. These measures were collectively coined the "immune risk profile" and have been adapted over the past decade to incorporate additional parameters. The continued fine-tuning of the immune risk profile is useful for determining the effects of regular exercise in the elderly. For example, it is generally accepted that middle-aged and elderly individuals who are habitually active are healthier, and evidence from cross-sectional studies shows enhanced immunity in physically active aging adults when compared to inactive counterparts. This evidence includes: (1) greater in vitro responsiveness of T cells to mitogens; (2) reduced frequency of antigen-experienced and aging T cells; (3) enhanced production of interleukin-2 and expression of T lymphocyte interleukin-2 receptors; (4) greater in vivo immune responses to vaccines and antigens; and (5) longer lengths of chromosomal telomeres in leukocytes.

As discussed in chapter 1, the average length of telomeres can differ significantly among individuals of the same age. However, numerous studies suggest that the length of telomeres is a heritable quality. To test this hypothesis, investigators have used white blood cells collected from monozygotic and dizygotic twins. The lengths of telomeres from monozygotic twins were similar, whereas the lengths of those of dizygotic twins were different. Significant correlations between the length of paternal telomeres and those of offspring telomeres were also observed. The lengths of telomeres can be modified by genetic and epigenetic factors, sex hormones, reactive oxygen species, inflammatory reactions, and physical activity. A critical minimum length indicates the arrest of the cell cycle or the aging of the cell. The immune system is sensitive to the shortening of telomeres because its competence depends on the renewal and expansion of T and B cells and other types of cells. Cells of the immune system are unique since they can up-regulate telomerase, the telomere-extending enzyme, and limit attrition of telomeres.

Experiments on the transplantation of hematopoietic stem cells reveal that they undergo aging and that their self-renewal capacity is also limited by the shortening of telomeres. However, investigators have observed successful aging of the active elderly whose functional immune cells have significantly shorter telomeres than those of the subjects' younger counterparts. Thus, it seems that one's length of telomeres and aging prospects are influenced by genetics, but that even those people with shorter telomeres can age successfully by being physically active. The innate component of the immune system is comparatively well preserved, though some age-dependent alterations are seen. In contrast, adaptive immunity deteriorates with aging primarily because of decline of naive T and B cells, as well as reductions in the absolute numbers of T and B lymphocytes.

It seems that one of the main problems of the aging immune system comes from a chronic imbalance between inflammatory and anti-inflammatory networks that favors pro-inflammation. Inflammatory responses correlate with age-related diseases and contribute to unsuccessful aging. As mentioned above, inflammaging is the age-dependent up-regulation of chronic viral infections and exposure to damaging agents. Environmental stress and inflammation link telomere shortening to oxidative stress. This includes intrinsic and extrinsic factors acting both on the whole organism and on the single cell. For example, it has been shown that smoking, low socioeconomic status, obesity, cardiovascular disease, and demineralization of bone are correlated with shorter lengths of telomeres. Aging-related oxidative damage of DNA bases (or single- and double-strand breaks) occurs more frequently in the elderly. This makes the broken ends of DNA molecules more resistant to repair and leads to aging via nontelomeric mechanisms. Oddly, successful aging is represented by nonagenarians and centenarians who exhibit better control over inflammatory responses.

Immunity, Influenza, and Aging

A number of years ago, one of my neighbors retired. Soon thereafter he and his wife and son moved to Las Vegas. My neighbor liked poker chips and told me he was moving to Las Vegas to collect them. He was a native of New Jersey and had spent his entire life in the Garden State. Shortly after arriving in the humidity-free state of Nevada, he contracted a respiratory illness. This hospitalized him and a few weeks later caused his death. His wife and son returned to New Jersey, but not to the home and neighborhood they had recently vacated.

After events like this and others like Hurricane Sandy, a "superstorm" in New Jersey and New York in October 2012, I have found myself wondering about regional airborne flora and fauna, the immune system, and disease and death. Arguably, animal and plant products that originate hundreds or even thousands of miles away can infiltrate living areas one has acclimated to. In addition, by relocating we can unwittingly become exposed to the indigenous airborne flora and fauna of our new atmospheric environs. In both circumstances, undetected airborne matter enters our bodies, aging or otherwise. Such foreign material can cause disease and death. Because of compromised immune systems, these influences are probably more common in the elderly than in the young. I noticed in the spring of 2013—the first growing season after Sandy—that my lawn had been invaded by several species of weed-like plants I had never seen before.

As my own body was acclimating to a new geographic environment (the Dallas–Fort Worth area, where I lived circa July 1, 1984 to July 1, 1985) and as the seasons changed, I occasionally woke up unable to breathe. These frightening respiratory events occurred between midnight and 2:00 or 3:00 A.M. and startled me out of my sleep. Fearing I would lose consciousness, I leaped out of bed, bent over, and gasped for air. Such bouts of impaired breathing came on unexpectedly once or twice every few weeks. I did not see a doctor but wondered if I was having asthma-like respiratory attacks, something I had never experienced before. I reasoned that something in the air I had previously not been exposed to was causing a respiratory allergic reaction and bronchospasms. I hoped that my immune system would adapt and that the experiences would end. They did, shortly after the first frost.

Normal immune function requires specific oxidative states. Reactive oxygen species are necessary for killing pathogens, limiting the specific immune response, and ending inflammation. Evidence of the involvement of reactive oxygen species in creating immunity comes in part from patients suffering from chronic granulomatous disease. This disease is caused by lack of a specific enzyme. Notably, the disease and the associated lack of reactive oxygen species lead to immunodeficiency and recurrent infections, including abscesses, pneumonia, and osteomyelitis. In response to stimulation, phagocytes of such patients do not generate reactive oxygen species. This is problematic for the person's defense because macrophages and neutrophils must generate reactive oxygen species to efficiently kill bacteria through phagocytosis. Fortunately, patients with this disease are able to produce another enzyme, called myeloperoxidase. This enzyme catalyzes the conversion of hydrogen peroxide and chloride ions into hypochlorous acid. Hypochlorous acid is much more potent than hydrogen peroxide (a reactive oxygen species) in killing bacteria.

In conclusion, bone marrow and its multitude of immune-related activities are compromised with longevity. Hematopoietic stem cells become less able to renew the circulating population of immune blood cells due to the shortening of telomeres and the accumulation of damaged DNA. Macrophages lose their bactericidal capacities and their numbers decrease. The number of antibody-producing B cells decreases, which leads to reduced affinity and diversity of immunoglobulins. The antigen-presenting function of dendritic cells decreases with age, causing profound changes in cellular immunity. And the homeostasis of lymphocytes is modified as fewer naive immune cells are created. Collectively, these changes lead to enhanced susceptibility to pathogens and to more serious outcomes of disease and injury.

5

The Aging Reproductive System

Conception and Aging

The reproductive systems of mammals, including humans, contain many of the intriguing mysteries of life. Under normal circumstances, fertilization of an egg by a sperm determines only the "genetic gender" of a zygote (the newly combined egg and sperm). About eight weeks later, the "physiological gender" begins to emerge. With few exceptions, the details of what happens biologically for the first eight weeks after conception are unknown. As almost everyone knows, however, the fertilizing spermatocyte must carry a Y chromosome in order for the genetic gender to eventually become a physiological male. The sex-determining region of the Y chromosome (SRY) is absent from the X chromosome. Without the SRY, the genetically programmed female becomes the phenotypical female (anatomically normal).

Still, in the first eight weeks after fertilization, male and female hormones and their corresponding receptor proteins play a major role in the morphological development of the zygote and its successors, the conceptus, embryo, and fetus. In the absence of adequate estrogen and progesterone receptors in the developing tissues, a genotypic female (XX chromosomes) might express, later in development, a more masculine phenotype. Similarly, a genotypic male, in the absence of the full complement of androgens and their corresponding receptors, could resemble the phenotypic female. Though not common, there are multiple disturbances to the normal male and female geno- and phenotypes.

I will leave the remaining details of this topic to the authors of books on inborn errors of metabolism and other congenital anomalies. However, considering what I have just written, we should all be amazed that the ratio of female to male births in the world throughout time—as far as we know— has been approximately 1:1. Moreover, the complicated chemistry should give the reader an added appreciation for the complexity of potential disturbances in this reproductive balance.

Except for the common cholesterol molecule found at the beginning of some elaborate biochemical pathways, female progesterone-like molecules are precursors to male androgen hormones. Similarly, female estrogen-like hormones rely on androgen precursors. Both genders carry both sets of hormones, and disruptions in the flow of chemistry can and do occur in the normal course of conception, development, and maturation. This, in part, explains the wide variety of differences in the appearances and behavior of males and females, from childhood through maturity.

Our discussion of the aging reproductive system will begin with the onset of puberty. Experts usually think of human aging as beginning in one's early twenties. However, no normal twenty-year-old thinks much about aging. I wasn't especially aware of my own aging until I was in my late thirties. I was at a gathering of my extended family in Lava Hot Springs, Idaho. A number of us had put on swimming suits and were preparing to tube down the Portneuf River. I remember looking at my chest and being surprised and annoyed to discover that most of the hair there was graying. If I had noticed this before, I certainly hadn't paid serious attention to it. I was angry and a bit embarrassed that my siblings and children would see. At the time I thought of myself as too young and too fit to have such an aged characteristic. After all, I naively thought, gray chest hairs were reserved for men in their seventies and eighties.

Now consider one or two of the current mysteries about the ovaries and testes, sites for the synthesis of adrenal-like steroid hormones. The female fetus possesses at twenty-nine weeks of gestation the greatest number of immature germ cells (oogonia) that she will ever have: approximately 6–7 million. This number declines to 2–3 million just before birth and to less than half a million at the onset of puberty. Why the marked decline? Conversely, the male testis ("testes" is the plural) does not begin producing spermatocytes (mature sperm cells) until puberty (which occurs at an average age of thirteen to fourteen years). The female, through atresia, loses eggs before birth and will stop producing them altogether at or near menopause, while she is still relatively young. Conversely, beginning at puberty the male is able to produce sperm cells throughout his mortal lifetime. Additionally, between about ages twelve and fifty-two, the average woman will ovulate only several hundred mature, fertilizable ova, while the average man produces hundreds of millions of sperm cells. What causes these marked and significant age-related differences in the genders? Why are the differences important?

To help us understand aging, scientists have learned more about telomeres. Telomeres are repeating DNA sequences at the ends of chromosomes that protect genes from the loss of nucleotides as cells divide. In the cells of our bodies telomeres shorten with age. This limits the number of times a cell can divide and thereby contributes to aging. Conversely, the length of telomeres increases with age in male germ cells. This means the offspring of older fathers inherit longer telomeres. Moreover, the lengthening of telomeres, predicted by each year that a father's or grandfather's reproduction is delayed, is equal to the yearly shortening of telomeres seen in middle-aged to elderly women. These modern genetic observations suggest a mechanism by which humans might extend late-life function as average age at reproduction is delayed within a lineage.

The Aging Male External Genitals

Disorders of sexual function are common among men of all ages, ethnicities, and cultural backgrounds. It has recently been estimated that in 1995 more than 152 million men worldwide experienced erectile dysfunction, and that this number will rise to approximately 322 million in 2025. Higher circulating plasma concentrations of testosterone appear to be associated with greater sexual activity in healthy older men, but not in younger ones. Furthermore, higher testosterone concentrations might shorten the latency of erection stimulated by exposure to sexual material, and testosterone replacement in males whose testes' function is reduced restores sexual interest (libido), shortens latency, and increases both the frequency and magnitude of spontaneous erections that occur during REM sleep. Similarly, withdrawal of androgen replacement therapy in hypogonadal males leads to a decline of libido in three to four weeks, and hypogonadal men who never receive the therapy have difficulty is achieving an erection.

For most males after puberty, nocturnal erections happen four to five times per night at roughly ninety-minute intervals, with episodes lasting thirty to forty-five minutes. The total time of nocturnal penile erections ranges from one and a half to three hours per night and accounts for about 25 percent of the total sleep time. Ninety percent of the episodes of REM sleep are associated with penile erections, with maximum changes in circumference of the penis and 70 percent of full rigidity. The number of episodes of erection and maximum erections decrease with age, from seven and four per night at age thirteen, to three and a half and about two per night at age seventy, respectively. As a result, total time of erections decreases by about 25 percent between these two ages. Interestingly, most dreams associated with nocturnal erections do not contain sexual content. Erections on waking usually represent events associated with the last episode of REM sleep and are not related to fullness of the urinary bladder.

Males reach peak sexual capacity in their late teens, and a steady decrease in sexual responsiveness occurs thereafter. Among other things, the decrease in responsiveness is characterized by prolongation of the time required to achieve full erection, the size and firmness of an erection, and the duration of an erection. With age, sustaining an erection requires continuous stimulation of the genitalia. Orgasm and ejaculatory sensations frequently become less intense as well. Loss of penile erection occurs more rapidly, and the refractory period—the time it takes to achieve a second erection following the first—becomes longer. The volume of ejaculate in men also decreases with age. Experiments in rodents have shown that advanced age is associated with decreases in the number of penile nerve fibers that produce the enzyme nitric oxide synthase. In humans and other mammals, nitric oxide synthase produces nitric oxide. Nitric oxide is a vasodilator, and penile erection depends on vasodilation. Also in aging rodents the maximum intracavernous pressure decreases. This pressure results from the volume of blood in the veins and related structures of the penis and is responsible for erections and rigidity. Similar information is not yet available for humans.

Cancer of the penis is another component of aging in men. Diego Rivera, a Mexican muralist, was also known for having multiple sexual partners (which we now know increases a man's risk of developing penile cancer, as explained below). He lived in a country where most men at the time were uncircumcised (another risk factor). After developing cancer of the penis, Rivera refused surgical removal of the organ. Instead, he traveled to what was then the Soviet Union for radiation therapy. He died a painful death from the disease and the side effects of his therapy.

The incidence of cancer of the penis in industrialized nations has to be viewed in the context of the high proportion of circumcised men living in them. In the United States, where two thirds of men are circumcised, the average age of men who first seek help for cancer of the penis and related conditions is sixty years. The typical distribution of ages of men with the disease is: 4 percent for men in their thirties, 14 percent for men in their forties and fifties, 22 percent of men in their sixties, and 31 percent of men in their seventies. The incidence drops to 12 percent for men in their eighties. Assuming an average life expectancy of seventy-five years, approximately seventy-five men out of every hundred thousand in the United States develop cancer of the penis. However, the disease occurs almost exclusively in uncircumcised men, so the chance of an uncircumcised man getting penile cancer would be higher—seventy-five men out of every 30,000, or one man in four hundred. It should also be pointed out that in the United States, men of Latino descent have the highest incidence of the disease, followed by black men and then whites and Asians.

The pattern described above is in marked contrast to patterns observed in women for cervical cancer. Human papilloma virus is an established cause of cervical cancer, and there has been immense progress in understanding the natural history of this viral infection in women. The virus's prevalence is highest in women eighteen to twenty-four years of age. It then decreases through middle age, after which it remains steady for the remainder of the life span. Human papilloma virus is the most common sexually transmitted infection in men and women in the United States, with an estimated 6 million new cases each year. There is now a growing interest in understanding the relationship between infection with the virus and disease in men, including the development of genital warts and cancer of the penis.

The consistently higher prevalence of human papilloma virus in men suggests that women have a stronger immune response against it. Across

all ages this is supported by studies of the plasma showing higher circulating concentrations of antibodies to the virus in women than in men. Once
a man contracts the virus, it takes an estimated six to twelve months and
rigorous therapy to eradicate the virus. However, this timing is influenced
both by age and by the number of female sexual partners the man has had.
Increasing age and lower numbers of female sexual partners are associated
with a greater probability of clearing an infection earlier. The converse is
also true.

Another effect of aging in men is that the foreskin of the penis
becomes discolored. This begins near the head of the penis (gland penis)
and progressively extends distally through the shaft. The discoloration can
leave the penis looking mottled. The phenomenon is related to the embryonic origins and physiological roles of genital skin fibroblasts. These
fibroblasts are crucial for the androgen-dependent development of male
external genitalia and the normal expression of androgen receptors and
5α-reductase. Some investigators have focused on the effects of testosterone and dihydrotestosterone on androgen receptors and transcription
of 5α-reductase II in cultured genital skin fibroblasts from pre- and post-
pubertal males. The investigators have found that there is no effect of age
on the actions of these male sex hormones on the development of androgen receptors or the corresponding enzymes. However, there is a significant decline in the enzyme's messenger RNA levels as men age. The
investigators concluded that the low levels of messenger RNA reflect their
insignificant role in the further maturation of external genitalia (such
fibroblasts are needed only before the age of four to five years).

Melanocytes are also importantly involved in the coloration of penile
skin. They are able to proliferate throughout a lifetime, but a stem cell
reservoir in hairless skin (such as the palms of the hands, soles of the feet,
and fingertips) has not yet been found. However, scientists have recently
shown that multipotent stem cells isolated from human foreskin lacking
hair follicles are able to migrate to the epidermis to differentiate into
melanocytes. These experimental dermal stem cells, grown in culture outside the body, displayed a capacity for self-renewal but did not express
markers typically found in melanocytes. In addition, cells derived from
single-cell clones were able to differentiate into multiple lineages, including melanocytes. These results demonstrate that stem cells in the dermis

of human skin can become mature epidermal melanocytes. This finding could change our understanding of the etiological factors in melanocyte transformation and pigmentation disorders.

Considering what I have written in the previous few paragraphs, it seems reasonable to conclude that married men who have limited their sexual activity over a lifetime to one woman are least likely to be affected by human papilloma virus and related sexually transmitted diseases. A similar conclusion might be drawn for women. John and Ann Betar (ages 102 and 98 years, respectively, in 2013) of Fairfield, Connecticut, were married in 1932. With family members, they celebrated their eighty-first wedding anniversary on November 25, 2013, Thanksgiving Day, in their home. The Betars were recognized in 2013 by the Worldwide Marriage Encounter as the currently living couple whose marriage has survived the longest in the United States. With a smile, John said he still drives Ann wherever she wants to go, and that the secret to success in marriage is to be forgiving, to not hold grudges, and to agree with whatever your wife says.

The Aging Testes

Recent studies, such as the Massachusetts Male Aging Study, have shown that between the ages of forty and seventy years, circulating plasma concentrations of both free (unbound to proteins) and albumin-bound testosterone decrease annually by about 1 percent in men. Decreases in circulating gonadal male hormones in both aging and obesity are caused by a parallel decline in the functional capacity of the hypothalamic-pituitary axis. Some observers have suggested that 90 percent of older men with reduced concentrations of testosterone show evidence of hypothalamic-pituitary dysfunction. This is reflected by low circulating concentrations of luteinizing hormone and its impaired release when the pituitary is stimulated by gonadotropin-releasing hormone. A decrease in the number of Leydig cells in the testes and in their release of testosterone in response to human chorionic gonadotropin in aging men has also been shown.

Leydig cells are the testosterone-producing factories of the testes. The cells develop from undifferentiated stem cells present in the testes of newborns. Four discrete stages in the growth of adult Leydig cells have been characterized: Leydig stem cells, Leydig progenitor cells, immature Leydig cells, and adult Leydig cells. Leydig stem cells are undifferentiated but are capable of infinite self-renewal (autogenesis), differentiation, and replenishment of their population. Leydig progenitor cells are derived from Leydig stem cells, are spindle-shaped, possess receptors for luteinizing hormone (from the pituitary gland), and are highly mitotic (self-dividing). They produce little testosterone but considerable quantities of testosterone precursors. Leydig progenitor cells give rise to immature Leydig cells, which are round, contain large amounts of smooth endoplasmic reticulum (protein synthesizing cellular machinery), and produce some testosterone but also have very high levels of testosterone precursors. A single division of these cells produces terminally differentiated adult Leydig cells that produce high levels of testosterone.

The decline in plasma testosterone mentioned above typically begins in the fifth decade of life and causes changes in body composition; energy balance; muscle strength; and physiological, sexual, and cognitive functions. The production of testosterone depends on the stimulation of Leydig cells by luteinizing hormone. Luteinizing hormone is intermittently secreted into the systemic circulation by the pituitary gland in response to another hormone or factor, gonadotropin-releasing hormone or factor. It comes from the hypothalamus. Testosterone and one of its enzymatically altered products, estradiol, then give negative feedback via the systemic circulation to the hypothalamus and pituitary gland to temporarily suppress the release of luteinizing hormone and production of testosterone. In response to these reductions, gonadotropin-releasing hormone and luteinizing hormone are again produced. This negative feedback cycle continues and results in the periodic release of luteinizing hormone, followed by the periodic production and secretion of testosterone.

In the second half of the twentieth century, investigators reasoned that the age-related decline in testosterone could be caused by a reduction in the number of functioning Leydig cells. To test their hypothesis, they studied brown Norway rats. This species lives to be older and is healthier than other strains of rat. Brown Norway rats typically die of heart disease at about forty months, gain little weight as they age, and rarely develop testicular, pituitary, or other tumors. Consequently, they are useful in distinguishing between age- and health-related deficiencies in endocrine and physiological functions. In these rats, reductions in testosterone result from the inability of aged Leydig cells to produce testosterone, not to a decline in the actual numbers of functioning Leydig cells—that is, Leydig cells simply become less efficient. As yet we are not certain if the same is true in aging humans.

The idea that exposure to oxidants is related to the deterioration of the Leydig cell's ability to synthesize protein and DNA has also been investigated. This seems to be a plausible explanation for two reasons. First, oxidants are produced during the synthesis of testosterone by the testes. Second, oxidants damage critical components of the steroid-synthesizing biochemicals. Some of the more damaging oxidants, also called reactive oxygen species, are superoxide anion, hydroxyl radical, and peroxynitrite. These and other oxidants, such as hydrogen peroxide, are produced as byproducts of steroid synthesis and might be responsible, at least in part, for age-related changes in functioning Leydig cells.

Following this line of reasoning, investigators have shown that contraceptive doses of testosterone administered to rats suppress release of luteinizing hormone and production of testosterone. Removal of testosterone-impregnated implants restores steroid synthesis in the Leydig cells of rats. This experimental approach reversibly suppresses the function of Leydig cells, forcing them into a state of so-called steroidogenic hibernation until the removal of testosterone-impregnated implants. It raises the possibility that long-term suppression of steroid synthesis might prevent or delay the aging of Leydig cells. To test the hypothesis, researchers tested the implants in rats of three or thirteen months of age (young and middle-aged). Eight months later, when the rats were eleven (middle-aged) and twenty-one months (old), the implants were removed, and the synthesis of luteinizing hormone was restored. Two months after that (rats were then thirteen and twenty-three months of age), Leydig cells were isolated and found to produce equivalent, high levels of testosterone. As expected, testosterone implants suppressed steroid synthesis. Two months after the implants were removed, Leydig cells from both middle-aged and old rats produced testosterone at the same high levels of young Leydig cells. Thus, by long-term suppression of steroidogenesis in rats, the reductions in testosterone that otherwise invariably accompany aging did not occur.

The mechanisms involved remain unclear, and whether these experimental results can be translated to humans is unknown. An attractive possibility, of course, is that long-term suppression of steroidogenesis prevents cellular damage by oxidants that are byproducts of testosterone synthesis. As yet there is no evidence that direct administration of oxidants can cause damage to Leydig cells, and whether such damage, if it occurs, might be involved in the aging of Leydig cells. These and related questions are under active investigation.

Confusingly, a few studies have shown the absence of correlation between erectile dysfunction and testosterone concentration. However, older men who have long-standing reduced function of the gonads usually complain of loss of sexual interest and activity, decrease in the volume of seminal emissions, loss of nocturnal and morning erections, and loss of energy and sense of well-being. And since testosterone replacement is associated with improved self-reported libido, sexual potency, and both subjective and objective measures of nocturnal erections, significant decline in testicular function is likely to be the primary cause of sexual dysfunction in aging men. The extent to which an age-related decrease in testosterone has direct consequences for physical or cognitive functions as well as for mood and overall quality of life, and the levels of testosterone at which these occur, remain uncertain, as does the role of testosterone supplementation.

The Aging Vas Deferens and Epididymis

The vas deferens is a tubular structure that carries mature sperm cells from the testes to the urethra. It is generally assumed that men who for congenital reasons lack a vas deferens have few or no sperm cells in the urethra but that the production of sperm is normal. Such men also tend to have smaller testes, possibly reflecting a reduced mass of testosterone-producing Leydig and other cells or a reduced extracellular matrix. Procedures for identifying this condition in young and old men include diagnostic biopsies, aspiration of the contents of the testes and epididymis, and other methods for extracting and quantifying the numbers of sperm cells. In one study, thirty-three men with congenital absence of the vas deferens underwent these diagnostic procedures; spermatogenesis was normal in all but four of them. Causes for impaired spermatogenesis included inflammation and pain caused by varicose veins in the gonads and other structures of the scrotum. Underlying genetic abnormalities were also responsible.

Other investigations have sought to determine changes in the chemistry of the vas deferens with age. Studies in laboratory animals have revealed variations in the neurochemical coding of nerve fibers to the testes. In one adult human study, investigators used immunofluorescence techniques to examine the distribution and patterns of colocalization of important chemicals, including neurotransmitters. The compounds of interest included neuropeptide Y, vasoactive intestinal peptide, calcitonin gene-related peptide, substance P, galanin, somatostatin, nitric oxide synthase, and the catecholamine-synthesizing enzymes tyrosine hydroxylase and dopamine beta-hydroxylase. In addition, an antiserum to vesicular acetylcholine transporter was incorporated to chemically tag cholinergic nerve terminals. Vas deferens removed at vasectomy from adult males ranging in age from twenty-eight to eighty-three years served as tissue samples. Results of this study provided evidence that changes occur in the neurochemistry of nerves innervating the vas deferens, and that this takes place sometime during puberty.

Immunostaining for protein gene products revealed a dense plexus of branching varicose nerve fibers throughout the smooth muscle coat of the human vas deferens. The smooth muscle coat is composed of a thin inner longitudinal layer, a much thicker middle circular layer, and an outer longitudinal layer. Regardless of age, the density of the intramuscular nerve fibers was similar in all specimens examined, and the majority of the specimens used protein gene products as general nerve markers. Such studies suggest that the muscle coat of the human vas deferens is richly innervated by autonomic nerves, the density of which does not appear to decline with advancing age. Most of the intramuscular nerves of the human vas deferens contain both tyrosine hydroxylase and dopamine beta hydroxylase and can therefore be classified as noradrenergic—that is, nerves that release norepinephrine as their main neurotransmitter. It is generally accepted that noradrenergic nerves are excitatory to the smooth musculature of the vas deferens. Thus the density of autonomic nerves in the human vas deferens is apparently not affected by age, unlike that reported in the urinary bladder, where innervation in elderly subjects is about half that of young adults.

Another structure, the epididymis, plays a fundamental role in the storage and maturation of sperm. To achieve full fertility of spermatocytes during the life span, epithelial cells of the epididymis undergo significant changes. From infancy to adulthood the tubular diameter, luminal diameter, and height of the epithelium increase markedly. Aging in the mammalian epididymis is also associated with a general decline in physiological functions, particularly fertility. The molecular basis of age-dependent development and decline of fertility is largely unknown, and the corresponding changes at the cellular and morphological levels in the epididymis from birth through old age are also poorly understood. Conversely, it is well established that a functional epididymis is dependent on testicular androgens, and that circulating androgens change significantly during the life span (see the discussion of testosterone and Leydig cells above). Therefore, during human male development the contents of testosterone in the epididymis reach a plateau at puberty and remain at a relatively high level until adulthood. Thereafter, remarkable cellular and histological changes take place during aging, accompanied by a decrease in the volume of semen and epididymally acquired sperm motility. Simultaneously, the proportion of abnormal spermatocytes increases, while the luminal diameter of the epididymis is significantly reduced and the height of epithelial cells in the wall increases.

In spite of the well-known importance of micro-RNAs as regulators of the expression of genes in many biological processes, an age-related, genomewide analysis of the expression of genes in the human epididymis did not take place until about 2010. Among other things, they discovered that the newborn human epididymis expressed the fewest mRNAs but the largest number of micro-RNAs, whereas the adult and aged epididymides expressed the most mRNAs but the fewest micro-RNAs, a negative correlation between mRNAs and micro-RNA during aging.

Among the specific genes found in the epididymis of newborns, the hemoglobin (Hb) gamma globin genes (Hbg1 and Hbg2) demonstrated the highest expression. This is consistent with previous reports showing that Hbg1 and Hbg2 are normally expressed in the fetal liver, spleen, and bone marrow. These two gamma globin chains, together with two alpha globin chains, constitute fetal hemoglobin, which makes up 50–95 percent of the hemoglobin in newborns. These findings reveal one more organ (the epididymis) that is capable of responding to the hypoxia of the uterine environment.

It is difficult to obtain normal human epididymal tissue samples, especially when trying to cover the range of ages that a study conducted by Chinese investigators did. So a weakness of that study is that only one sample was analyzed for each age (there were no replications or statistical analyses). Doubtless as more tissue samples become available, future studies will be expanded to allow a more in-depth analysis.

Changes in the physiology of reproductive and sexual activity and body composition and mental performance in the aging male cannot be ascribed simply to a decline in the function of the testes as defined by low circulating concentrations of testosterone and growth hormone. Structural changes in organs at different regulatory levels, such as reduced mass of neurons in the hypothalamus, also play a role. In addition, increased circulating concentrations of luteinizing and follicle-stimulating hormones can be observed in old men. In these men in general, endocrine functions are sufficient to maintain fertility because, except for sperm motility, quantitative and qualitative measures of the functional capacity of semen are not affected by age. Nevertheless, as in all other physiological functions, there is considerable individual variability in the properties of the hypothalamus, pituitary gland, and gonads. This variability is both necessary and sufficient to explain differences in male reproductive function with age.

In summary, the male reproductive system can be viewed as an interactive homeostatic network in which changes at different levels occur during aging. Depending on their origins—that is, the hypothalamic pulse generator, the anterior pituitary gonadotropes, or the steroid-producing cells in the testis—these changes can result in the loss of circadian rhythmicity and the alteration of plasma concentrations of testosterone and other hormones. Still, such changes in aging men are not as pronounced as those associated with menopause in women. Thus, much research has focused on changes in growth stimulating and inhibiting factors that change with age. In the field of male reproductive physiology, there is still much work to be done.

Reproductive and Sexual Aging in Women

Everyone knows that women outlive men. Of the world's centenarians and supercentenarians, about 90 percent are women. The explanations for this vary, and there are no definitive data to tell us why women outlive men. Regardless, the female reproductive axis (hypothalamus, pituitary gland, and ovaries) is unique in that it reaches an aged state when other organs in the woman's body are generally healthy. The process that depletes the supply of eggs (oocytes), which begins before birth and ends with menopause, cannot be predicted precisely by chronological age because its time of onset varies widely among women. Still, there are time-lines called clinical staging systems to help with this uncertainty (table 5–1). These make it possible to estimate where a woman is in her process of reproductive aging. Such systems are based on patterns of menstruation and are better predictors than chronological age. And staging is useful because it provides a way to attribute the symptoms of a woman during this time to changes in the perimenopausal state. Staging can also help predict the time to final menstrual period, and it can identify potential risks to health. There are now well-described symptoms that are linked to specific time points along the menopausal transition (table 5–1 and similar data). Moreover, evidence is building that at least some menopausal symptoms not previously attributed to the deficiency of estrogen can be successfully treated by exogenous hormones.

As American women age, 30–50 percent of them complain of sexual dysfunction. Aging, menopause, and declines in circulating concentrations of estrogen, progesterone, and testosterone significantly increase the incidence of sexual complaints. Evaluation of physiological components of the female sexual response has been technically challenging and difficult to standardize. Moreover, it is somewhat dependent on a woman's connectivity to her spouse. Regardless of the length or nature of a male and female relationship, its quality is enhanced by emotional intimacy, autonomy without too much distance, ability to manage stress, and the maintenance of a positive perception of self and the relationship. To understand and treat the effects of aging on sexuality, it is important to address the three components of sexual desire—drive, beliefs and values, and motivation—as well as the social context of a woman's life. It is also essential to understand how the physiological changes in female as well as male sexual functioning affect desire. Other health-related changes that occur with aging must also be recognized and addressed.

TABLE 5-1

Staging Systems Used to Help Define Perimenopausal States in Women

STRAW[a] definition		PENN-5[b] definition		ReStage[c] definition	
Premenopause (Stages −5 to −3)	Regular cycles, with no change in cycle length	Premenopause	Regular cycles, with no change in cycle length	Premenopause	Regular cycles, with no change in cycle length
Early transition (Stage −2)	1 cycle length change (≥7 days)	Late premenopause	1 cycle length change (≥7 days)	Early transition	1 cycle length change (≥7 days)
		Early transition	≥2 cycle length changes (≥7 days)		
Late transition (Stage −1)	2–11 months of amenorrhea	Late transition	3–11 months of amenorrhea	Late transition (0.85 probability of FMP[d] within 5 y)	Ages 45–49 y: 60 days—11 months of amenorrhea; ages 40–44 y: at least 60 days of amenorrhea +60 days of amenorrhea within the next 10 bleeding segments
Postmenopause (Stage +1, +2)	≥12 months of amenorrhea	Postmenopause	≥12 months of amenorrhea	Postmenopause	≥12 months of amenorrhea

Source: L. Butler and N. Santoro, "The Reproductive Endocrinology of the Menopausal Transition," *Steroids* 76 (2011): 627–35. [a]Stages of Reproductive Aging Workshop. [b,c]Attempts subsequent to STRAW to further define the stages of late amenorrhea. [d]Final menstrual period.

Recently investigators have developed methods for evaluating physiological and subjective components of the female sexual response in the clinical setting. They have also determined the effects of age and estrogen status on these components. For example, in one study forty-eight women with complaints of sexual dysfunction were investigated clinically and physiologically. Measurements included peak velocity of genital blood flow during systole, vaginal pH, intravaginal pressure-volume changes (compliance or distensability of the vagina), and perceptions of genital vibration (stimulation). Subjective sexual function was assessed using a questionnaire. Measurements were repeated and the questionnaire retaken under baseline conditions and following sexual stimulation. Age was then correlated with both physiological and subjective responses.

Genital stimulation resulted in increased blood flow, increased vaginal compliance, and increased vaginal pH in all women. Older women (ages fifty-five to seventy-one) and postmenopausal women not on hormone replacement therapy had significantly reduced physiological responses. Their baseline subjective complaints were higher when compared with younger women, including low arousal (67 percent), low desire (21 percent), difficulty achieving orgasm (92 percent), and pain or discomfort during and/or following intercourse (67 percent). Thus, with aging many women can expect to be less sexually active. This can affect relationships, especially if the woman's partner is still sexually active and desires intimacy. Of course, there are other ways to express intimacy beyond genital intercourse; moreover, aspects of relationships go well beyond the sexual and have little or nothing to do with age. These include communications and finances. If a husband and wife have never had good communications, then they should not expect to feel more connected as they age. Similarly, if they did not agree on how to manage their money when they were younger, they should not expect their sexual relationship, as far as it is affected by finances, to improve with age.

The Aging Ovaries

Each woman is endowed with a population of oocytes during fetal development. At about sixteen weeks after conception, the two ovaries combined contain several million oocytes (undeveloped eggs). This population of oocytes is surrounded by a layer of protective cells called the granulosa, which helps define the primordial follicle pool. At any chronological age, more than 99 percent of a woman's eggs are present as nondividing, non-growing primordial or primary follicles. At birth, only 1 or 2 million primordial follicles remain. The loss (atresia) during the second half of fetal development is due to apoptosis, or so-called programmed cell death. Atresia is the periodic process by which immature ovarian follicles (potential future eggs) degenerate and are subsequently resorbed during the follicular phase of the monthly menstrual cycle. After birth, the high rate of follicular atresia declines, so that at menarche (one's first menses, or menstrual cycle) approximately 400,000–500,000 primordial follicles remain. The continuing decline during the reproductive years causes the numbers to drop below 1,000 at the time of menopause.

Thus, in women the reproductive aging process is characterized by a gradual decrease in both the quantity and quality of oocytes. It is nearly impossible to directly measure the number in humans. This is not true in other animal species, and extrapolations from them to humans have been made. Before the beginning of the twenty-first century, the only estimates of numbers of primordial follicles across the human female reproductive life cycle were drawn from several older studies, using combined data. Those investigations concluded that the rate of oocyte decline follows a biphasic pattern. At about thirty-eight years of age, as women move toward menopause, there is a distinct acceleration of decline. After menopause the decline slows. More recently, investigators have used stereological techniques and found that although the total oocyte counts at any particular age were similar to what previous researchers had found, the decay in the number of primordial follicles was best described by a simple power function, with no biphasic change in the rate of decay. Rather, the more recent investigations have found a consistently increasing rate of follicular atresia as women age.

The age-related decrease in the number of follicles dictates the onset of irregularity in the menstrual cycle and its cessation. The parallel decay in oocyte quality contributes to the gradual decline in fertility and the final occurrence of natural sterility. Typically, about twenty follicles mature each month but only one, the dominant follicle, is ovulated. The remaining follicles undergo atresia. No one knows how one follicle becomes dominant among many thousands of developing follicles. Nor do we know the details of what initiates apoptosis among the remaining, nondominant follicles. Similarly, as a woman ages we do not know if the follicles that she ovulated in her thirties and forties were healthier or less fertile than those that she ovulated in her teens and twenties. After all, the former follicles will have spent ten to thirty more years in the ovaries than the latter follicles. We do know, however, that after ovulation the remaining components of the single dominant follicle become a corpus luteum (light-absorbing body). This residual follicle plays an important role in the latter half of the monthly ovarian cycle. For example, it secretes progesterone in response to luteinizing hormone, which helps suppress further development of the remaining follicles. In both males and females, luteinizing hormone is essential for reproduction. An age-related decrease in the female's physiological ability to reproduce has distinct implications in view of the current trend in Western societies to postpone childbearing. Older women have a greater probability than younger women of producing offspring with congenital impairments. Menopause is the final step in the process of ovarian aging.

In females, luteinizing hormone supports another population of specialized cells in the ovary: theca cells, which provide androgens and hormonal precursors for the synthesis of estrogens including estradiol. At the time of menstruation, follicle-stimulating hormone initiates follicular growth that specifically affects granulosa cells. With the rise in estrogens, luteinizing hormone receptors are also expressed on the follicle, which causes it to produce more estradiol. Eventually, when the follicle has fully matured, a spike in the production of estrogen by the follicle initiates a positive feedback loop in the hypothalamus that stimulates the release of luteinizing hormone from the anterior pituitary. This increase in the production of luteinizing hormone, called the LH surge, lasts for twenty-four to forty-eight hours and triggers ovulation. It thereby not only releases the egg from the follicle but also initiates conversion of the residual follicle into a corpus luteum that, in turn, produces progesterone and prepares the uterine lining for the implantation of a fertilized egg (the zygote). Luteinizing hormone is necessary to maintain luteal function for the first two weeks of the menstrual cycle. If pregnancy occurs, the circulating concentrations of luteinizing hormone decrease and so do the physiological processes it supports. Luteal function is maintained by human chorionic gonadotropin, a hormone similar to luteinizing hormone but secreted from the new placenta.

Release of luteinizing hormone at the pituitary gland is controlled by pulses of gonadotropin-releasing hormone from the hypothalamus. The pulses of this hormone, in turn, are subject to estrogen feedback from the gonads. In the male, luteinizing hormone acts on the Leydig cells of the testes and is responsible for the production of testosterone, an androgen that exerts both endocrine and intratesticular activity during spermatogenesis.

The Aging Uterus and Related Structures

The uterine wall also shows the effects of aging on reproductive tissue. The inner wall and lining of the uterus, made up mostly of visceral smooth muscle and connective tissue, is called the endometrium. Each month before ovulation during a woman's menstrual years, the endometrium thickens and becomes denser. This is due to storage of blood and nutrients in preparation for the possibility of fertilization and implantation of a fertilized egg. When implantation does not occur, the stored blood and other tissues of the thickened endometrium are shed, the uterine wall becomes thinner again, and the monthly uterine cycle begins once more (women's monthly reproductive cycle can be subdivided into the menstrual cycle, ovarian cycle, uterine cycle, and perhaps others). As women age and become peri- and postmenopausal, the uterine wall becomes even thinner, as the uterus loses visceral smooth muscle mass. Moreover, the uterus is normally held in place inside the pelvic girdle by various muscles, ligaments, and other soft tissues that also lose mass with age. Sometimes, because of childbirth or difficult labor and delivery earlier in life, these muscles and other soft tissues weaken. As a woman ages and with the natural loss of the hormones of the reproductive years, her uterus can collapse into the vaginal canal, causing a condition known as uterine prolapse. Muscle weakness or relaxation can allow the uterus to sag into and even protrude out of the body via the vagina.

Uterine prolapse can be divided into several stages. First-degree uterine prolapse is when the cervix droops into the vagina. During second-degree uterine prolapse, the cervix adheres to the opening of the vagina. In third-degree uterine prolapse, the cervix extends or protrudes outside the vagina, and during fourth-degree prolapse the entire uterus is outside the vagina. The latter condition is called procidentia. Other conditions are also associated with uterine prolapse. For example, cystocele (or a hernia-tion or bulging) of the anterior vaginal wall, in which part of the urinary bladder presses against the vagina, may lead to symptoms of overactive bladder (that is, it may affect urinary frequency, urgency, retention, and incontinence). Enterocele (or herniation of the posterior vaginal wall) is when part of the small intestine presses against the vagina. Under these conditions, standing leads to a pulling sensation and backache. These symptoms are relieved only when lying down. Rectocele (or herniation of the lower posterior vaginal wall causes the rectum to press against the vagina. This makes bowel movements difficult to the point where a woman might need to push on the inside of the vagina to empty the bowel. The above conditions can require corrective surgery.

In the 1990s hormone replacement therapy in postmenopausal women attracted national and international attention. I had a female grad-uate student at the time. A married woman who had raised two sons, she had decided to return to the university to earn a PhD. This nontraditional graduate student expressed an interest in the effects of endocrine hormones on the heart and coronary circulation of mammals. Part of the reason why estrogen replacement therapy was then an intriguing topic was because of estrogen's hypothesized coronary vasodilator capacity and women's heart disease.

My student obtained some of the more frequently prescribed hor-mone replacement drugs, and we began studying them in experimental animals. One of our objectives was to be more rigorous than the current medical literature had been in quantifying their coronary vascular effects. Using a careful experimental design, my student discovered that the drugs had no coronary vasodilatory properties at all. Instead, the drugs induced both intermittent and sustained coronary vasoconstriction, reduced blood flow to the heart, and in some cases caused ventricular arrhythmias. Her results did not complement the medical wisdom of the day, so she began presenting her findings at national conferences and publishing them in peer-reviewed scientific and medical journals. A further sign of confusion about the drugs was that about half of the gynecologists in the United States who were themselves postmenopausal were taking hormone replacement therapy (and prescribing it to their patients), but the other half were not. What a mixed message these physicians were sending to the perimenopausal female population about their future choices.

Since that time, the effects of hormone replacement therapy on reproductive function and genital vascular hemodynamics in aging women have been steadily investigated. The aim of one study was to measure clitoral artery blood flow with and without the therapy. Doppler sonography was performed in twenty-five postmenopausal women who were about forty-five to fifty-five years of age and who for about two years had been using a combined hormone replacement therapy (0.625 milligrams of conjugated equine estrogens, my student's drug of choice for investigation, plus 2.5 milligrams of medroxyprogesterone acetate, daily). Thirty-five postmenopausal women of the same age who had not used the therapy served as a control group. Peak systolic flow velocity in the clitoral artery, resistance to blood flow, and the pulsatile nature of flow were measured. Peak systolic flow velocities were modestly but significantly higher in women on hormone replacement therapy (15 ± 5 and 12 ± 5 centimeters per second, respectively). These clinicians concluded that hormone replacement therapy, under the conditions of their investigation, improves blood flow to the clitoris and that evaluation of clitoral blood flow is a potential tool for assessing the effects of hormone replacement therapy in postmenopausal women.

The Aging Breast

Breasts are glands, and the aging process in the breast concerns some women who in their twenties and thirties see their mothers' breasts begin to lose shape, sag, and droop. However, this concern is not limited to younger women seeing changes in their aging mothers. Aging women themselves are probably the most likely to be affected by such changes. The female breast is composed of lobes and lobules, ducts and ductules, connective tissue and interstitium. Ptosis of the breast is the medical term for drooping or sagging female breasts and is a natural consequence of aging. The causes of drooping and sagging breasts were unknown until recent years. Investigators are finding that the primary culprits of sagging over a woman's lifetime are cigarette smoking (which destroys elastin of the breast and chest wall, which supports the position of the healthy breast), changes in body mass index (cyclic gain and loss of weight promotes sagging), the number of pregnancies a woman has had (a direct correlation to sagging), and breast size before pregnancy. The drooping of breasts with age is also influenced by genetic makeup (which is the primary determinant of a woman's skin elasticity) and the balance of adipose and glandular tissue. Plastic surgeons categorize the severity of ptosis by evaluating the position of the nipple relative to the inframammary fold (the point of attachment between the lower margin of the breast and the thorax). In the most advanced stages, the nipples are well below the fold and point toward the ground. The opposite is true in cases of more successful aging (in which there is less sagging and nipples remain above the fold and projecting forward). Both the density of the breasts and the elasticity of the skin affect the ratio of less-dense fat to more-dense mammary glands.

Other than the factors listed above, the biggest contributor to sagging of the breasts appears to be age. Unless cosmetic, reconstructive surgery is undergone, breasts sag with age, and the degree of sagging is semiquantifiable using categories such as the following:

Grade I: mild ptosis—the nipple is at the level of the inframammary fold and above most of the lower breast tissue.

Grade II: moderate ptosis—the nipple is located below the inframammary fold but higher than most of the breast tissue.

Grade III: advanced ptosis—the nipple is below the inframammary fold and at the level of maximum breast projection.

Grade IV: severe ptosis—the nipple is far below the inframammary fold and points toward the floor.

Pseudoptosis—the nipple is located either at or above the inframammary fold, while the lower half of the breast sags below the fold. This is most often seen when a woman stops nursing because her milk glands atrophy.

Parenchymal maldistribution—the lower breast tissue is lacking fullness, the inframammary fold is very high, and the nipple and areola are relatively close to the fold. This is usually a developmental anomaly.

When the aging breast is examined through an electron microscope, details begin to emerge. The most noticeable change is the gradual decrease in size of lobules with age. In addition, the proportion of lobular epithelium increases, while the contents of fibrous and connective tissues decrease. When these changes are quantified, however, one finds that the volumes of connective tissue and epithelium reach their maximum capacity during the third decade of life and then decline rapidly. The ages at which such changes and menopause occur indicate that involution of breast tissue begins well before menopause.

Other than size, no significant structural changes in the shapes of lobules occur with aging. The normal lobular profile is slightly elliptical, and the three-dimensional lobular shape is more ellipsoidal than spherical. A notable finding in one study was the relative absence of changes indicative of fibrosis or mammary dysplasia in any of several age groups studied (the subjects were ten to eighty years of age). The true incidence of such changes in the normal breast is difficult to assess accurately, since it is impossible to distinguish the earliest disease-related changes from those caused by age alone. Enlargement of the ducts is considered a normal feature of the aging breast. Atypical and dilated lobules often found in cancerous breasts seem to represent distinctive lesions that are unrelated to the normal changes of aging. They are usually indicative of imminent or already apparent changes that are associated with disease.

Cancer of the breast is something that concerns most women but is not limited to them. Men experience cancer of the breast as well, although not at as high rates as women. While I was revising the current chapter a close friend, about ten years younger than me, had a tumor removed from his right breast. He had completed four biweekly rounds of chemotherapy and was on his third or fourth round of biweekly radiation treatment. Just like women, this friend lost his hair, his appetite, and about fifteen pounds during the treatment. His oncologist told him that rapidly replicating cells would be most affected by the chemotherapy and radiation. These included residual tumor cells and cells of the hair follicles and mucosal membranes (such as those lining the oral/digestive spaces). My friend described food as being bland or completely tasteless. He was in near-continuous systemic pain following each round of chemotherapy, and the oncologist monitored his white and red blood cell populations throughout the therapy. This friend, like most other men and women I have known who have been exposed to chemo or radiation therapy, looked and acted washed out and wasted during the ordeal.

The Aging Skin

The skin is composed of several layers, with the outermost layer (epidermis) composed mainly of dead cells. Intrinsic aging of the dermis (which lies beneath the epidermis) affects mainly the interstitial spaces and extracellular matrix. In the skin the amount of elastin and collagen decreases with age, and their protein structures change. As a result, the skin becomes stiffer, less malleable, and more vulnerable to injury. Aging also reduces the number and function of sweat glands and the secretions of nearby sebaceous glands. This makes the skin drier and causes it to look more wrinkled as we age. Aging also reduces the content of melanocytes in hair follicles, resulting in graying of the hair, spotting of the skin, and reducing of skin tone (color). A related condition that affects women more than men is sagging skin. As women lose muscle mass, particularly in the triceps and biceps, and accumulate adipose in the subcutaneous tissues (which lie between skin and muscle), they can develop flabby arms.

Some women are so self-conscious about their flabby arms that they avoid wearing short-sleeved clothing. Onset of flabby arms can be delayed and even markedly attenuated by certain kinds of exercise. It is also affected by the diet they follow from an early age. Doing push-ups regularly (even from the knees instead of the toes) and lifting of free weights several times per week are helpful. The earlier in life one begins these practices, the more effective they are. You do not need expensive exercise attire or wasteful memberships to gyms. A few sets of dumbbells (for example, pairs of weights each weighing five, ten, and twenty pounds), a bench, and a little space such as a spare bedroom will do the trick. As with most of life's worthwhile activities, determination, discipline, and consistency are key ingredients. Of course, depending on your particular body morphology, it is possible to overdo the weight training. Women who tend to be either endomorphic or mesomorphic can develop biceps that look decidedly masculine.

A deficiency of estrogen, among other things, reduces the thickness of an aging woman's skin and its immune defense mechanisms, resulting in greater infestation by microbes and pathogens. Susceptibility to mechanical injuries and chemical irritations also increase with age, and healing of the skin after an injury slows. Menopause further attenuates the cell-mediated immune response to microbes and allergens, and the skin of the female external genitalia is a case in point. The morphology and physiology of the vulva and vagina change over a lifetime, and the most salient changes are linked to puberty, the menstrual cycle, pregnancy, and menopause. At birth, the vulva and vagina exhibit the effects of residual maternal estrogens, and during puberty these tissues acquire mature characteristics. Interestingly, there has been a recent trend toward the earlier onset of puberty, particularly in Western young women, and the trend is stronger in blacks than in whites. The vulva and vagina further adapt to the needs of pregnancy and delivery, but after menopause, tissue atrophy ensues.

Postmenopausal changes in the functions of skin barriers, skin hydration, and susceptibility to irritants have been observed on exposed skin and the vulva. For example, older women with incontinence are at increased risk for developing dermatitis of the vulva. A combination of factors, such as tissue atrophy, skin hydration, limited mobility, and lower capacities for tissues to regenerate, increases the risk of morbidity from incontinence dermatitis in older women. Moreover, more women than men are concerned about their aging skin, especially their facial appearance. This is particularly true about wrinkles around the eyes and mouth (so-called crow's feet). This concern explains, in part, the multibillion-dollar annual skin care and cosmetics industries.

In the skin of women and men there are two kinds of aging, intrinsic and photo. Intrinsic aging occurs at sites that are not regularly exposed to the sun, such as the buttocks. In contrast, photo aging results from long-term exposure to the sun's ultraviolet radiation. Skin not exposed to the sun shows minimal signs of aging. Skin exposed to the sun, such as the face, shows the greatest effects of aging. As skin ages intrinsically, it thins, more in the dermis (for example, the dermis loses about 20 percent of its thickness) and less in the epidermis. The outermost layer of the epidermis, the stratum corneum, changes very little with age. The rate at which keratinocytes develop slows with age, but the aging cells remain in the stratum corneum longer, which explains why this layer does not thin with age. Two other cell types in the epidermis also decrease with age: the melanocyte population (cells that give pigmentation to the skin; reduced photo protection results from reduced melanocytes) and Langerhans' cells (Langerhans' cells are part of the skin's immune system; reduced density of these cells reduces immunity).

If you are aging in the southwestern United States, your skin probably looks several years older than that of your aging counterparts in the northeastern part of the country. This is explained, in part, by excessive exposure to the sun, the increased heat, and the relative lack of humidity in the Southwest versus the Northeast. As a rule, the skin of people in the Northeast is well hydrated compared to that of people in the Southwest. Thus, photo aging increases the natural effects of intrinsic aging and causes wrinkles that would occur minimally or not at all because of intrinsic aging alone.

In June 2014 my wife and I took and extended road trip through the Southwest and West. As we left the Dallas–Fort Worth area and passed through West Texas (Abilene, Midland, El Paso), then northwest through New Mexico and Arizona, our nasal mucosal membranes became dehydrated, dried and cracked. We camped near Carlsbad and Alamogordo, New Mexico, when daytime temperatures were 110–115° Fahrenheit. Considerable effort was required to keep sufficiently hydrated during the rest of our road trip to compensate for the arid effects of the Southwest.

Also, it is never too early or too late to consider the effects of diet and eating habits on aging. Although this topic is more appropriate in a chapter on the gastrointestinal system, a word of warning is fitting here. In spite of what I have just written and contrary to popular opinion, one should never use exercise and working out as a way to control body weight. Exercise should be used only to build muscle mass, tone existing muscles, and minimize the rate of muscle loss with aging. One's weight and size can only be controlled through diet. If you overeat by consuming 3,000 calories in one day, then undereat by consuming fewer than 2,000 calories in the next day or two, that will quickly compensate for the difference. Remember, weight accumulates one gram at a time (goldfish by pretzel, mouthful by mouthful, and gulp by gulp). Weight is also lost one gram at a time by reducing the volume and quantity of what you eat and drink. Discipline at the table and during mealtimes is the key to controlling one's weight and appearance, for both women and men. And as my son's preschool teacher taught the children, you are what you eat from your head to your feet.

6

The Aging Urinary System

Kidneys and Glomerular Filtration

Most healthy people have two kidneys. The kidneys are located on either side of the abdominal aorta or vertebral column (thus, they are bilateral organs) and lie outside of the abdominal cavity. Because of this location, they are called retroperitoneal organs. In healthy adults, kidneys are bean-shaped structures, are supplied with blood by the left and right renal arteries, and weigh about 125–175 grams in men (and 10 percent less in women). Kidneys have many physiological responsibilities, including: (1) maintaining the composition and osmotic activity of body water; (2) filtering blood and maintaining its homeostasis by assisting in the long-term regulation of blood pressure and blood volume; and (3) helping the lungs regulate the acidity and alkalinity of all body fluids.

The structural and functional unit of the kidney is the nephron. Each kidney has about one million nephrons (plus or minus a few hundred thousand). Nephrons consist of both blood vessels and tubules. Blood-borne materials are filtered out of the blood vessels at a structure called Bowman's capsule. The specific sites of filtration are the glomerular capillaries, which are tucked neatly inside Bowman's capsule. Bowman's capsule gives rise to the renal or urinary tubular system. Downstream from a Bowman's capsule, many filtered products are moved from the tubules to the peritubular capillaries. Products that do not get reabsorbed in this way, including water and solutes, accumulate inside the tubules. Tubules from several adjacent nephrons drain their contents into a single collecting duct. The contents of the collecting ducts are delivered to the renal calyses and renal pelvis and eventually make their way through the ureters and into the urinary bladder. The bladder's contents are stored until urination.

Water and solutes that get filtered at the glomerular capillaries are called ultrafiltrate, glomerular filtrate, or glomerular ultrafiltrate. The composition of the ultrafiltrate inside a Bowman's capsule is similar to that of plasma, except that the protein concentration is lower. Any product in the ultrafiltrate that does not get reabsorbed by peritubular capillaries is ultimately eliminated as urine. Peritubular capillaries make up a second capillary network that is found downstream from and works in conjunction with the upstream glomerular capillaries. During any twenty-four-hour period, the kidneys are continually challenged by varying states of body hydration (hyperhydration, dehydration, and normohydration), fluctuations in blood pressure, the changing acidity of body fluids, and the need to eliminate byproducts of metabolism (such as urea). Theirs is not an easy job.

In an evaluation of kidney function, the physiologically most useful variables are renal clearance (removal of a substance from the plasma), glomerular filtration rate (GFR), effective renal plasma flow (ERPF), and filtration fraction (FF—that is, GFR divided by ERPF). Accurately assessing these variables usually requires hospitalization. This is because blood vessels must be catheterized, drugs are administered (injections and continuous infusions), and blood and urine samples are collected. All this exposes the patient to invasive procedures and the possibility of infections. Reliable evaluation of kidney function using the above variables (as well as collecting magnetic resonance images [MRIs] and other images) is important for a variety of reasons, including: (1) assessing the effects of treatment; (2) adjusting the doses of drugs; (3) determining function in potential kidney donors; and (4) answering questions such as those about the effects of aging and gender on kidney function.

Between the ages of twenty and fifty, human males have greater values for GFR, ERPF, and FF than females do, but when the values are normalized for body surface area (which is 1.70–1.90 square meters in adult humans), no differences exist between the genders. Also when normalized, relative values for GFR, ERPF, and FF decline between the ages of twenty and fifty in men but not in women. After age fifty, these differences between the genders disappear. In contrast to mice and rats, in humans the female reproductive hormones were thought to protect women against cardiovascular disease and some forms of cancer in the premenopausal years, but such protection is probably lost after menopause or never occurred at all (see chapter 5).

Declining Renal Function with Age

As already mentioned, kidneys filter the blood and dispose of wastes and excess fluid as urine. A decline in kidney function can begin in one's twenties and thirties and is a significant concern in older adults. In men there is an age-related decrease in the number of nephrons (glomeruli, blood vessels, and tubules). This change might not appear in women until they are in the peri- or postmenopausal state. Loss of glomeruli results in decreased filtration and impairments in other kidney-mediated homeostatic processes. This is a problem because as we get older and become less healthy, we take more medications. If the mass of functioning renal tissues has declined, blood might not be adequately filtered and cleared of the potentially harmful byproducts of these medications. The medications and their metabolic byproducts can then accumulate to toxic levels. This is one reason why close attention must be paid to medications with warnings that include, for example, wording like "caution in patients with renal insufficiency or kidney disease." Moreover, some medications are known to hasten the age-related decline in kidney function. These include nonsteroidal anti-inflammatory drugs, certain antihypertensive drugs, and some medications for diabetes.

Our kidneys also regulate the concentrations of electrolytes and minerals in the body fluids, such as calcium, chloride, bicarbonate, potassium, and sodium. In a state of good health, the circulating concentrations of these electrolytes are in balance with concentrations in spaces surrounding blood vessels and inside cells. When disturbances occur, the kidneys manage them. For example, the kidneys eliminate excess potassium through excretion in the urine. If the kidneys are impaired by age or disease, potassium can accumulate in the circulation and tissue spaces. This is called hyperkalemia. The heart, nerves, and other tissues are extremely sensitive to excess potassium. For example, a doubling of physiological concentrations of potassium (from 4 to 8 milliequivalents per liter) can cause cardiac arrhythmias (heart palpitations). A tripling or quadrupling of potassium might lead to cardiac arrest and sudden death. It is not generally known that hyperkalemia, among other constituents of the injectate, is used to cause death by lethal injection. It causes cardiac arrest.

The kidneys are also responsible for maintaining the homeostasis of sodium. Significant increments or decrements in sodium are both detrimental to normal physiological function and good health. For example, the concentrations of sodium in body fluids markedly influence the volumes of those fluids. This is one way that excess dietary sodium contributes to elevated blood pressure. As the concentration of sodium inside blood vessels increases, so does the corresponding volume of water. Wherever sodium is, water follows. The expansion of water inside ever-stiffening blood vessels (because of the loss of vascular compliance with age) can lead to marked elevations in blood pressure. Also, as aging occurs the kidneys' hormonal response to dehydration is impaired. Kidneys lose their ability to conserve both salt and water when these physiologically essential elements of a healthy life should be retained. This results in older adults being vulnerable because their kidneys cannot concentrate the urine to conserve body water.

Another disorder that results from gradual kidney dysfunction with age is anemia. Anemia results from a reduction in the number of circulating red blood cells and/or a reduction in the hemoglobin content inside the red blood cells. In defining anemia, the World Health Organization's criteria are the gold standard: <12 grams of hemoglobin per deciliter of whole blood for women and <13 for men. The kidneys produce a hormone called erythropoietin (EPO), which stimulates the production of red blood cells in bone marrow. Erythropoietin concentrations measured in young adults are strikingly similar across studies. Not unlike other physiological measures in elderly populations, erythropoietin concentrations for older subjects are extremely variable.

What happens to the circulating concentrations of EPO with age is an important question. What is the potential effect of gender on EPO is another. When the production of red blood cells decreases, so does the blood's ability to carry oxygen, which leads to hypoxia (inadequate oxygenation of the tissues). Hypoxia explains, in part, why so many elderly people who are in poor health are tethered to small oxygen tanks. Because of impaired respiration, circulation, and/or hematology, they cannot get enough oxygen from the atmosphere. Therefore, these patients must get the gas from the higher partial pressures of compressed oxygen in cylinders.

Signs and symptoms of anemia-induced hypoxia to watch for in your aging loved ones include fatigue, weakness, and pale skin color. A simple blood test can reveal if one's red blood cell concentration, hemoglobin concentration, and hematocrit have decreased. Significant decrements in one or more of these important variables reduce the oxygen-carrying capacity of the blood—which, for optimal health, should be maintained at near twenty milliliters of oxygen for each hundred of blood.

The Baltimore Longitudinal Study of Aging (BLSA) describes patterns of changes in circulating concentrations of EPO and hemoglobin and in diseases that complicate kidney function with age. The BLSA is an intra-mural research program within the National Institute on Aging. Initiated circa 1958, this project has produced results that have contributed greatly to our understanding of physiological changes that occur with normal aging. Healthy volunteers aged twenty and older are enrolled in the study and participate in follow-up visits approximately every two years. Currently the study has about 1,500 active participants.

Accumulating data from the BLSA reveal that with age, increased production of erythropoietin is necessary for the maintenance of circulating concentrations of hemoglobin. The data also show that this compensatory mechanism is less efficient in people with diabetes or hypertension, who show a diminished response to anemia-mediated elevations in erythropoietin. In addition, people who are at increased risk of developing anemia later in life—for example, those who will have diabetes or hypertension—have higher levels of erythropoietin under baseline conditions in their young adulthood. Data from the BLSA also suggest that even when EPO concentrations are within the normal range, a high-normal EPO concentration in a young or middle-aged nonanemic adult might be a warning sign of evolving glucose intolerance (diabetes) or hypertension, a notion that warrants further investigation.

Investigators of the BLSA have drawn two novel conclusions. First, in patients who do not develop anemia, higher levels of EPO are required to sustain normal hemoglobin concentrations as a person ages. This may be due to an increased resistance or diminished responsiveness of the EPO-sensitive progenitor cells to EPO. Second, in people who develop anemia, some processes interfere with the production and/or release of erythropoietin to sustain a normal hemoglobin concentration. Studies in aged mice have also demonstrated a diminished erythropoietin response to anemia or hypoxia. Thus, an increased production of erythropoietin with age has been described. It has been proposed that in some individuals this is not sustainable and accounts for or contributes to the development of anemia.

Several mechanisms could account for an inadequate erythropoietin response in older people. Disturbances in the regulation of cytokines might reduce the production of erythropoietin or the responsiveness of bone marrow to it. Alternatively, age-related fibrosis of the renal interstitium, without a corresponding change in glomerular filtration, could diminish production of EPO by influencing the physiological point at which it is released. Finally, some investigators believe that aging is associated with diseases such as diabetes or hypertension that are known to impair the function of renal tubules. A combination of aging and disease might attenuate the renal release of erythropoietin.

In mammals, 80–90 percent of the kidney's nephrons are found in the renal cortex, the outer region of the kidney. Only 10–20 percent of the nephrons are found in the renal medulla, or inner region. The renal microcirculation serves the nephrons and includes renal afferent and efferent arterioles, as well as glomerular and peritubular capillaries that the arterioles supply blood to. From experiments in female mice, there is evidence that the mass of the smallest cortical renal blood vessels decreases with age. Female mice and women also lose estrogen with age. To compare the effects of aging and the loss of estrogen on these vessels in female mice, one group of investigators studied young (six months) and aging mice (eighteen to twenty-two months). In the oldest mice, the density of blood vessels was reduced to about one-third of that in the young mice. Removing estrogen from young mice (by surgically removing their ovaries, a procedure called ovariectomy) was not responsible for the loss of density of microvessels. This was demonstrated by replacing estrogen in half of the mice whose ovaries were removed. There were no significant differences in the density of microvessels in the latter two groups— that is, the ovariectomized mice with and without estrogen replacement.

Similar results have been found in aging rats. One group of investigators discovered that there was no difference in age-dependent glomerular

atrophy between young or old intact male and female rats, and that neither ovariectomy nor estrogen replacement affected glomerular mass in
females. Conversely, hypertrophy of the tubular interstitium was greater in
old males than in old females. Results suggested that ovarian hormones do
not influence these aspects of kidney aging, and that the proliferation of
tubular interstitium is caused by being male. Also, when compared with
young male and female rats, old male rats had greater quantities of two key
enzymes in the renal cortex: nitric oxide synthase-3 and nitric oxide syn-
thase-1. Nitric oxide synthases are proteins that help mediate normal
growth, development, and function of the kidneys and other tissues and
organs. The contents of these enzymes in the tissues were preserved with
age in intact females (but with lower contents than in males), and ovariectomy did not affect this. Nor did replacement of circulating concentrations
of estrogen elevate the enzymes, suggesting that estrogens are not primary
regulators of renal nitric oxide synthases with aging in females. Conversely, the production of proteins that attenuate the actions of nitric
oxide synthase increase in aging male rat kidneys, compared with those of
females.

On Tuesday, August 21, 2012, about 11 A.M., I received an unexpected
telephone call. It was from my former dentist, who had retired about a year
earlier. During the thirty-six years that he treated me, we had become good
friends. I regretted his decision to retire but understood it. In the phone
call he described a close personal friend whose kidney health had recently
and precipitously declined. My former dentist asked permission to give his
friend my name as a potential source of information. I agreed. Fifteen minutes later that friend called. He is a semiretired physician living in San
Francisco. He has lived an active lifestyle (swimming and biking about
twenty minutes each per day), was diagnosed with leukemia in 2011, and
had surgery for the condition in December 2011. Between January and April
2012, he spent time in London and in Pittsburgh, and for about thirty days
he followed a diet that included mushrooms, which his wife had recently
researched. He was also taking medications with known renal side effects.

Prior to surgery, this man's circulating concentrations of creatinine
were 1.3 milligrams per deciliter of blood (mg/dL), which is about normal
for a healthy person his age. After surgery, his trips to London and
Pittsburgh, the medications, and the mushrooms, his creatinine

concentrations rose to 9.0 mg/dL. His corresponding estimated glomerular filtration rate (eGFR; estimated kidney function) was less than 40 percent. At the time of his telephone call, this man had been on kidney dialysis for several months, had had a kidney biopsy, and was diagnosed with interstitial nephritis. He wondered about the cause of his renal failure and was ascribing it to everything from diet and medications to a chronic bacterial infection dating back to 1986.

I empathized as I listened. What a quandary! How could he possibly rule out any of the above causes? Before offering any comments, I made it clear to him that I am not an expert in renal physiology, medicine, pharmacology, diet, bacterial infections, or the treatment of leukemia and interstitial nephritis. He understood but still sought my opinion. He asked if he could send me copies of his medical records, and I agreed. In exchange, I asked his (and my former dentist's) permission to tell this story. They agreed. The friend's medical records confirmed his telephone conversation but could not be used to rule out the possible contributions of his travels, recent changes in diet (mushrooms), leukemia, medications, or past bacterial infections as causes of his then-current dilemma.

Clearance and Kidney Function

Kidney function is properly assessed in the clinic by nephrologists and urologists who understand the kidneys and who are familiar with concepts such as renal clearance (see below) and its relation to the kidneys' ability to filter. Today, the relationships between circulating concentrations of creatinine and glomerular filtration rate are used more commonly to estimate GFR. Creatinine is a byproduct of muscle metabolism. Its rates of production and excretion remain relatively constant each day over many years. The constancy of these rates results in circulating plasma concentrations of creatinine, in nondiseased states, of about 1.0–1.5 mg/dL.

Because evaluating GFR using creatinine is not as invasive as classic, historic methods such as inulin (not to be mistaken for insulin; inulin is a plant product of the Jerusalem artichoke that can also be manufactured synthetically) clearance, plasma creatinine is rapidly becoming the gold standard for clinically assessing renal function. In a healthy young person, muscle mass does not change appreciably over a period of a few decades (for example, between the ages of twenty and forty-five). Of course, there are exceptions to this, such as purposeful bulking up in a gym. However, even in healthy men and women, muscle mass begins to decrease rapidly after the mid-forties. Thus, using circulating concentrations of creatinine to estimate GFR is fine during the early decades of adulthood. This is the time to establish a baseline for GFR that can then be used as one ages and one's health begins to deteriorate.

In order to assess the removal of a solute from the plasma (clearance of, for example, glucose, urea, or creatinine), one must be able to measure that solute in the plasma and in the urine. Historically, the marker of choice for assessing renal function via the principles of clearance has been inulin. To estimate clearance and the rate of glomerular filtration using inulin, it has to be administered to the body. This was done by renal physiologists first in experimental animals, then later in humans.

Clearance of inulin is considered a valid measure of renal function because inulin meets all the criteria that renal physiologists established for understanding and applying the following principles. Because of its small molecular size, inulin is freely filterable by the glomerular capillaries (criterion number one). Because of its chemical nature, including the fact that it is not metabolized by the kidneys, inulin is easily quantified in body fluids, including plasma and urine (criterion number two). Inulin is not reabsorbed, secreted, or stored by renal tubules (criteria numbers three through five). Finally, inulin is physiologically inert—that is, it has no known effects on the kidneys, such as altering renal blood flow (criterion number six). Thus, the amount of inulin excreted in the urine equals the amount filtered from the blood. With a few simple mathematical equations, including consideration of the six criteria just mentioned, clearance of inulin can be quantified. By manipulating those equations and employing the law of the conservation of mass, clearance of inulin becomes an acceptable physiological expression of GFR and therefore of renal function.

In addition to the above, clearance can be thought of as the virtual volume of renal arterial plasma, and its corresponding concentration of a solute, needed to account for the solute excreted in the urine. The rate of excretion of any solute, X, is the concentration of X in the urine times the rate of urine flow. Mathematically, excretion of X looks like this: ($U_x \times V$, expressed in milliliters per minute). The virtual volume of plasma and its corresponding concentration of X are expressed as (P_x) (RPF_a). RPF_a is the rate of renal arterial plasma flow, or the volume of flow delivering X to the glomerular capillaries. P_x is the concentration of X in the renal arterial plasma. According to the law of conservation of mass, these two expressions (the excretion and virtual volume of X) can be brought together as: $(P_x)(GFR) = (U_x)(V)$. Solving for GFR, we rewrite the equation as GFR $= (U_x)(V)/(P_x)$.

With the growing concern of medicine for infections caused by invasive procedures, use of inulin to determine renal function via clearance has become mainly an experimental procedure because the urethra, a vein, and an artery must be catheterized to perform this methodology, and the patient must be hospitalized. Therefore, naturally occurring (that is, produced by our bodies) substitutes for inulin have been sought. As mentioned earlier, by measuring circulating concentrations of creatinine, the clinician can estimate a patient's GFR with a considerable degree of precision. As long as muscle mass and daily activities (including filtration and urination) remain relatively constant, circulating concentrations of creatinine will remain constant (about 1 milligram per 100 milliliters of plasma).

Beginning about age twenty-one, GFR in a healthy adult male weighing seventy kilograms is around 125 milliliters per minute, or 180 liters per day. Glomerular filtration rate is modestly lower in healthy adult females, unless normalized for body weight or body surface area. Most of the filtered volume is water. Of the 180 liters that are filtered each day, all but 1.5 liters are reabsorbed by the kidneys. These 1.5 liters represent the average volume of urine excreted each day. However, as we age and begin to lose muscle and renal mass, circulating concentrations of creatinine can change. Moreover, acute renal failure as well as chronic nephritis, such as established and permanent inflammation of the kidneys, can markedly impair renal function. When the filtering capacity of the kidneys is impaired, clearance of creatinine and any other marker of GFR and overall renal function decrease. As this occurs, the circulating plasma concentrations of creatinine increase.

To minimize problems like those described earlier by my former dentist's friend, interested readers should be examined by a physician once or twice a year. The examination should include a blood work-up, for which you may have to go to a laboratory. It is best to have blood withdrawn when you have not consumed food or liquids (except adequate volumes of water) for eighteen to twenty-four hours. This is when your body is in what medical professionals refer to as an effective state of fasting.

An analysis of withdrawn venous blood can reveal several things about a person's renal health. For example, for the past ten or so years, my annual blood reports have included the acronym eGFR. As already pointed out, this stands for estimated glomerular filtration rate. Glomerular filtration rate is an expression of the adequacy of one's collective nephrons to produce a volume of ultrafiltrate that is normal for that person's gender, age, size, and other conditions.

The Aging Urinary Bladder

How can one tell if a urinary bladder is functioning properly or not? The bladder is located between the filtering kidneys and the urethra. It is a storage organ that is under both voluntary and involuntary neural control. Urine passes intermittently from the kidneys through two ureters into the lower body of the bladder and is stored there until one determines to release it by urination. If we are perceptive, we can learn how to recognize the earliest sensations telling us we need to void, as well as when the bladder feels full and it is suddenly urgent that we void. Bladder function can be tested in the clinic by an experienced urologist.

A clinical technique called cystometrography is used for evaluating bladder function and the physiological state of the urination reflex (also called the micturition reflex). A cystometrogram is a measure of the changes in muscle tone and bladder pressure as an empty bladder is incrementally filled to capacity. Tone is defined as the relationship between pressure inside the bladder (intravesical pressure) and volume of urine stored there. A clinician can determine this pressure- volume relationship by first inserting a catheter into the urethra, advancing it to the bladder, and using the catheter to empty the bladder. Once the bladder is empty, the clinician then records the intravesical pressure while filling the bladder, in increments of fifty milliliters (mL), with sterile water or saline solution warmed to room or body temperature. This procedure is intended to simulate filling of the bladder by the intermittent passage of urine through the ureters. The volume of fluid stored inside the bladder is the independent variable. Intravesical pressure is the dependent variable.

Increasing the volume of an empty bladder from 0 to 50 mL produces a rather steep rise in pressure. This means that during the initial change in volume the bladder wall is not very compliant. Continuing to increase the volume from 50 to 300 mL yields almost no further change in pressure. During this stage, the bladder is most compliant and is said to be filling passively. The high degree of compliance is thought to be due to the active relaxation of visceral smooth muscle (in the bladder wall) as the bladder is filled. At volumes greater than about 400 mL, additional increments produce marked elevations in pressure, and the bladder once again becomes noncompliant. The maximum capacity of the bladder in a seventy-kilogram adult is an estimated 550–650 mL. At such volumes, the person feels extremely uncomfortable, and the need to urinate is beyond urgent. In the nondiseased bladder, the patient first feels the urge to urinate at a volume of about 150 mL. He senses bladder fullness and the necessity to void at a volume of about 400–500 mL.

In a nonclinical setting and until a socially acceptable time and location are available, the central nervous system in a learned reflex inhibits the micturition reflex. This reflex is coordinated from the brainstem in a region of the pons called the pontine micturition center. The person voluntarily avoids emptying the bladder until reaching the appropriate time and place. Once he or she decides to urinate, the external urinary sphincter, which is made of skeletal muscle and is under one's volitional control, relaxes. Once this voluntary relaxation occurs, it is followed closely by relaxation of the involuntary, internal urinary sphincter. The latter sphincter is composed of visceral smooth muscle. When the sphincters relax, a small volume of urine moves from the body of the bladder into the posterior urethra near the neck of the bladder (the junction between the bladder and urethra). Mechanical stretch receptors in that region are stimulated and send sensory nerve signals to the pontine micturition center (and higher brain centers), telling them to stop inhibiting motor nerves that innervate the bladder wall. Once the motor nerve inhibition is withdrawn, those nerves release neurotransmitters that cause contraction of the bladder wall. The central nervous system continues to inhibit contraction of the sphincters, and a series of self-regenerating contractions and relaxations of the bladder wall empties its contents.

Benign Prostate Hyperplasia and Overactive Bladder

With aging, benign prostatic hyperplasia (BPH) or overactive bladder (OAB, more common in women) can upset the micturition reflex and one's daily patterns of urination. Also, damage can disrupt function. For example, spinal cord injuries that result in loss of voluntary control of the micturition reflex are often accompanied by retention of residual volumes of urine after micturition and corresponding bacterial infections. These can be frequent because the residual urine serves as an incubator for bacteria, which are always present. BPH and OAB can and do have pronounced impacts on lifestyle and one's interactions with other people.

Benign prostatic hyperplasia is a noncancerous enlargement of the prostate that restricts the flow of urine from the bladder. It is the most common disorder of the aging prostate and is the most frequent diagnosis by urologists for male patients ages forty-five to seventy-five. In eight of ten men, symptoms relating to changes in patterns of urination suggest BPH. Half of men in their fifties and 80 percent of them in their eighties have some symptoms of the disorder. Symptoms include frequent need to urinate, sudden need to urinate, interrupted sleep to urinate, need to strain or push on the bladder to urinate, difficulty beginning to urinate, pain or burning during urination, sensations of an incompletely emptied bladder after urination, and a weak or dribbling stream during urination. Approximately 8 to 9 million men between ages of fifty and eighty in the United States are candidates for treatment of BPH.

There are two periods in a man's life when the prostate enlarges. The first is during puberty, when it doubles in size. Then, near age twenty-five, the gland begins to grow again, this time more slowly. Years later this secondary growth results in BPH. During the latter growth phase, the prostate can double to quadruple in size, growing from an average volume of about 25 mL to 50–125 mL. The enlargement compresses the urethra and neck of the urinary bladder like tightening a clamp on a garden hose (the prostate surrounds the urethra). Upstream of the constriction, in the garden-hose analogy, the volume of water increases and the hose expands. With time, the overextended hose (stretched bladder) loses its elasticity and fails to revert to its original size and volume after the water (urine) is released. Downstream of the constriction, the flow of water (urine) is unusually slow. The extra-urethral compression and partial emptying of the bladder cause many of the symptoms of BPH.

Subjective outcomes for identifying the severity of age-related BPH can be assessed using the American Urological Association Symptoms Index (AUASI). This is the English version of the International Prostate Symptoms Score (IPSS), a measure often reported in European studies. The AUASI has been shown to have greater reliability than more objective measures such as monitoring the peak rate of urine flow. It is a self-administered test consisting of seven questions. The sum of the scores on the seven questions reflects the overall severity of the patient's BPH (0–7 is mild; 8–19, moderate; 20–35, severe).

Men are ineligible for the AUASI and IPSS tests if they are at high risk for urinary retention. This is defined as a peak urinary flow rate of less than 4 mL per second, or a residual volume after voiding of more than 250 mL. They are also ineligible if they have a history of prostate cancer, have had surgery for BPH, have urethral constriction or an overactive bladder caused by nerves, have a circulating plasma creatinine greater than 2.0 mg/100 mL, have had a prostate-specific antigen (PSA) concentration of more than 4.0 nanograms (ng) per mL of urine, are using medications known to affect urination, or have had a severe concomitant disease. Men over the age of forty-nine years who have had moderate-to-severe symptoms of BPH (an AUASI score of eight or more) and a peak urinary flow rate of less than 15 mL per second are also ineligible.

For any man who suspects he might be getting BPH but has not yet been diagnosed, a disciplined home test can be helpful. It will require careful observations for a few weeks and the purchase of some inexpensive equipment (500 mL graduated beaker, a 250 or 500 mL graduated cylinder, and a stopwatch—all of which can be purchased through Fisher Scientific, VWR, or other online vendors of medical supplies). You should also keep a log (daily, weekly, or monthly) of the amount of urine excreted. These simple tools and their consistent use will help you monitor patterns of urination. Later, the log will become useful as you explore the condition with your physician or urologist and consider taking medication and having a biopsy or surgery.

The first step in the self-administered home study is to keep a written record of your estimated levels of hydration and dehydration. For example, noting after breakfast, lunch, and dinner whether you are excessively hydrated (which could be marked in the log as "+++"), well hydrated (++), hydrated (+), modestly dehydrated (−), dehydrated (−−), or excessively dehydrated (−−−). This is important because the need to urinate and the rates of urine flow are first and foremost directly proportional to your state of hydration. If you are severely dehydrated, you urinate seldom or not at all. If you are excessively hydrated, you urinate frequently. Additional notes of your patterns of urination will be helpful (low, medium, and high volumes). Second, when you feel the urge to urinate at home, go to the bathroom with the pieces of equipment described above, your pencil, and your log. Urinate into the graduated cylinder or beaker, then record the rate of urination in mL per second. The best way to do this is to start the stopwatch (or follow the second hand on your wristwatch) when you begin urinating and stop it when you have finished. If you are an average adult and your bladder contains about 300–400 mL of urine, you should be able to eliminate most if not all of it in about 15–20 seconds. If you do not have mild to moderate BPH, your urine flow rate could be equal to or greater than 15 mL per second. If you have moderate to severe BPH, your urine flow rate could be less than or equal to 8 mL per second.

An example might be helpful. Imagine that the volume of urine collected at one voiding is 350 mL. Also imagine that you eliminated this in 15 seconds. Dividing 350 by 15 equals 23 mL per second. As mentioned above, a warning sign of BPH is a urine flow rate of less than 15 mL per second. In this example you can probably conclude that you do not have BPH but are simply overhydrated. You should repeat this simple test a few times each day for several weeks. It is important to keep track of the times of urination (e.g., 6:15 A.M. and 10:45 P.M.). There is a daily, physiological rhythm that affects kidney function, including the rates of filtration and excretion of urine. We urinate less in the late P.M. to early A.M. hours and more in the late A.M. to early P.M. hours.

Suppose your routine is to retire at 10:00 P.M. and get up at 7:00 A.M. In recent years you have found that if you don't drink some water or any other liquid before going to bed, you wake up during the night with a dry mouth and a strong sense of thirst. So you have established the practice of drinking a large glass or two of water between the hours of 6:00 and 10:00 P.M. As a result, you could be getting up several times in the late P.M. to early A.M. hours to eliminate the excess water. This is normal and probably has little to do with BPH. However, if you don't consume that much water between 6:00 and 10:00 P.M. but are still getting up two or three times each night, you might suspect that you have BPH. Once you have collected a few weeks' worth of data, average the results and let the outcome help you decide whether you need to see your physician or a urologist.

A second self-help test is to observe the color of your urine. It is best to do this by collecting all voided urine in your graduated beaker (500 mL). You should not try to estimate the hue by watching the stream of flow as it passes into the toilet or urinal. This is deceptive. The goal for urine coloration is to avoid extremes. Deep orange or yellow hues accompanied by low rates of flow are indicators of dehydration: drink some water. Conversely, nearly clear urine corresponding with high rates of flow is a sign of hyperhydration: reduce your consumption of water during the next few hours. Aim for a consistent coloration that avoids extremes. Achieving this goal will take discipline, practice, and patience.

During a twenty-four-hour period the average adult should consume about 2,500 mL, or about two and a half quarts, of water in all its forms—direct, indirect, and intrinsic. Direct water is what you drink straight out of the tap. You get indirect water from the coffee, tea, alcohol, soda, and juices you consume. Intrinsic water is found in fruits, vegetables, and all other food products we eat. The 2,500 mL from all three sources matches the volume of water we lose each day. We lose water through excretion (in urine and stools), evaporation (through the skin and in sweat), and respiration. It makes physiological sense that we should consume only the same volume of water that we eliminate. This is not only true of water but also of calories. If more of us practiced both principles there would be less obesity and sickness and greater health and contentment in the world.

Beyond self-help tests and a person's symptoms, BPH in the aging man can be diagnosed by a professional using a combination of approaches. First, a digital rectal exam allows the physician to palpate a small portion of the prostate through the wall of the rectum. Based on several exams over a few years, your physician can tell if your prostate is enlarging. Second, results from the AUASI or IPSS surveys, discussed above, are helpful. Third, the PSA blood test has been used for some time, although it remains controversial (medical insurance companies as well as other opponents have proposed its official discontinuance). PSA is a protein produced selectively by the cells of the prostate gland. If the gland is enlarging, then there are more cells producing PSA and its circulating concentrations should rise. PSA concentrations in a healthy thirty-five-year-old man should be about 1.0 ng/mL. This might increase slowly to 2.0 ng/mL by age fifty-five. If thereafter the number increases in a year or two to 5.0 ng/mL or more, there is cause for concern. And fourth, a study of the rate of urine flow and/or the use of rectal ultrasound, fifth, can confirm or disprove digital rectal diagnosis. Once BHP has been diagnosed, there are several options for treatment.

Nonsurgical and Minimally Invasive Treatment of BPH

I have stated above that many men in their forties through eighties have BPH, while few of those in their twenties and thirties do. Of course, many of us become more comfortable financially after age forty. This is a time when we begin to have more disposable cash and to gain extra pounds. For men, some of the extra weight is found inside the abdominal cavity. For women, it is more often carried on the thighs and buttocks. We see the protruding bellies, larger waists, bigger hips, and triple chins, but we do not often think about the internal effects of our obesity. They are there, however. For example, fat accumulates around the vocal cords and related structures, which contributes to sleep apnea and snoring. Peri- and intra-abdominal fat collects on the liver, gut, reproductive structures, and bladder. Conceivably, some of these fat depots invade tissues of the prostate gland, helping enlarge it.

Therefore, before you consider drugs and surgical treatment for BPH or OAB, try shedding excess weight—twenty or thirty pounds, or even more if needed. Don't try to do this through exercise. Rather, try eating smaller portions, consume less of the wrong and more of the right foods, and stop snacking. Once you've lost the weight, add an exercise routine to your improved discipline. Losing weight will not harm your prostate or adjacent urinary or reproductive tissues. In fact, by eliminating some of the fat content of these organs and tissues, their overall size could decrease, thereby relieving your symptoms. If there is no change in symptoms after you have lost weight, be assured that your overall health has still improved. You can confirm this with regular measurements of blood pressure, blood sugar, and circulating lipids (such as triglycerides and cholesterol).

To begin the above activities, make a record of your symptoms before losing weight. Then, during and after dropping the extra pounds, take additional notes. Compare the three sets of data and corresponding symptoms of BPH or OAB as you progress. Determine if things have improved. If they have, then you should be motivated to keep those extra pounds off. If they haven't, then you have ruled out one possible contributor (overweight) and can now consider other options (such as drugs and surgery).

Psychological anxiety has long been cited as a possible contributor to urinary tract problems. Emotional distress is one of the main activators of sympathetic nerves. Having regular and heated disputes and arguing with anyone are such stressors. Experimental results associating diastolic blood pressure and circulating concentrations of cortisol with BPH and OAB support an effect of psychological stress on the prostate and bladder, and there are a number of plausible mechanisms. Stress-related hyperactivity of the sympathetic nervous system decreases the rate of cellular apoptosis, which results in increased numbers of aging cells in the prostate. The administration of epinephrine and norepinephrine (fight-or-flight chemicals) causes contraction, hyperplasia, and hypertrophy of the prostate. Inhibiting the binding of these neurotransmitters to their receptors causes increased cell death and reduced proliferation in the prostate. Likewise, surgical severance of the sympathetic nerves that innervate the prostate decreases its size.

Conversely, norepinephrine blockers (also called alpha blockers) can also relax the ureters, thus interfering with the wavelike peristaltic contractions that push urine through the ureters and into the bladder. In the presence of norepinephrine blockers, urine can potentially accumulate in the ureters, overstretch them, and contribute to their loss of elasticity, tone, and physiological function. Another adverse side effect of norepinephrine blockers is postural hypotension, dizziness, and fainting. Postural hypotension is a drop in arterial blood pressure when a person rises from a sitting, prone, or supine position to an upright one. This is exaggerated when alpha blockers prevent vessels from constricting in response to increased blood volume (causing pooling of blood in peripheral veins and reducing flow to the brain and so forth). Fatigue, nasal congestion, erectile dysfunction, and abnormal ejaculation are all additional side effects of alpha blockers.

Over 90 percent of prescriptions for BPH are herbal medicines, especially saw palmetto extract (SPE). Saw palmetto is used by over two million men in the United States for the treatment of BPH and is commonly recommended as an alternative to drugs approved by the Food and Drug Administration (FDA). The use of SPE is discouraged by American clinicians and academicians because evidence of its benefit is inconclusive and because the FDA rejected SPE for the treatment of BPH for the same reason. In one double-blind trial, investigators randomly assigned 225 men over the age of forty-nine years who had moderate-to-severe symptoms of BPH to one year of treatment with SPE (160 milligrams twice a day) or a placebo. The primary variables monitored were changes in the scores on the AUASI and maximal urinary flow rate. Secondary outcomes included: (1) change in prostate size; (2) residual urinary volume after voiding; (3) quality of life; (4) laboratory tests including PSA; and (5) the rate of reported adverse effects. There were no statistically significant differences between the SPE and placebo groups in the change in AUASI scores, maximal urinary flow rate, prostate size, residual volume after voiding, quality of life, or serum PSA levels during the one-year study. The incidence of side effects was similar in the two groups. In this study, SPE did not improve symptoms or objective measures of BPH.

Research has proven that minimally invasive treatments for BPH can be safe and effective. Such approaches might be appropriate for persons who don't want to take daily medication for the rest of their lives but do not want to expose themselves to the risks of invasive surgery. Minimally invasive treatments include radio frequency therapy, interstitial laser coagulation, and transurethral microwave therapy. There are flaws with each of them, not the least important of which is the penetration of the walls of tubular structures through which the surgical instrument is passed (for example, the wall of the urethra or of the rectum). Radio frequency therapy delivers low-level energy through the urethra via a dose-controlled delivery system to destroy a well-defined (a misnomer) region of the enlarged prostate. Transurethral microwave therapy relies on the passage of microwaves through the wall of the urethra in an attempt to reduce the size of the prostate. Interstitial laser coagulation depends on the ability of a high-energy laser ray to destroy interstitial spaces and extracellular matrix in hopes of reducing the mass of prostate tissue. Reducing extracellular matrix does not reduce the numbers of PSA-producing cells (use of interstitial lasers). In radio frequency therapy, shields are supposed to protect the urethra from heat damage, and the procedure is indicated for the treatment of symptoms in men over the age of fifty with prostate sizes of 20–50 cubic centimeters. When compared with transurethral microwave therapy for resection of the prostate, the procedure improves the flow of urine and relieves symptoms of BPH with significantly fewer side effects. The procedure can be performed in a doctor's office using local anesthesia. Of the side effects the most common include obstruction of the flow of urine, bleeding, pain and discomfort, feeling an urgent need to urinate, increased frequency of urination, and urinary tract infections. Symptoms of BPH usually begin improving within two to six weeks if these side effects are not present. If they are, the efficacy of the procedure is of questionable value.

Invasive Treatment of BPH

There is a growing number of surgical options for treating BPH. These range from removing the entire prostate (total or radical prostatectomy) to removing the sections of it that are most problematic. However, such surgical procedures can stimulate regrowth and proliferation of remnants of a cancerous prostate that were not completely removed during the surgical procedures complicating the initial problem. Transurethral resection of the prostate, a more moderate procedure, is a surgical method in which a resectoscope is inserted into the penis and advanced through the urethra to the area of the enlarged prostate. The cutting tip of the surgical blade mentioned above must be passed through the wall of the urethra to gain access to the prostate. Then, by the process of surgical electrocautery, areas of enlargement are reduced by the combination of cutting (with a small surgical blade) and searing (passing an electrical current through the blade). This is the most common surgical treatment, and it requires spinal or general anesthesia and a stay of one to three days in the hospital. Catheterization of the bladder after the procedure is also required for several days. Adverse effects have included incontinence, impotence, retrograde ejaculation (which occurs when ejaculate flows upstream instead of downstream), infection, and loss of blood volume. Following is an excerpt from a patient who opted for transurethral resection to treat BPH.

For the past year or more I've had a real slowdown in my urine stream. I went on Flomax and was fine for about a month until all symptoms returned. My physician referred me to a urologist who discussed options and I opted for the green light laser surgery (where they vaporize the bladder neck to enlarge the opening). My outpatient surgery went fine, I removed the catheter the next day and had pain urinating, but it was bearable. My only instructions were to take it easy for two days. So within four to five days I was resurfacing my driveway, cleaning my garage, and not restricting my physical activity at all. At my two-week check up I still had blood in my urine but the urologist didn't seem concerned. Then a few days later my morning urine was pretty red. I went on-line before going to work and discovered that I should have taken it easy for two weeks rather than two days. After taking it real easy for a week my urine has been amazingly clear for three days. I have a real issue with the doctor for not warning me, but I'm lots better now because I figured out what to do.

Catheterization of the urethra for any reason can cause problems that were not present before the procedure. The urethra, like all tubular conduit organs (including all blood vessels except capillaries), is lined with endothelial cells. These important cells have a host of critical regulatory functions. Passing a catheter through such a structure (en route to the prostate or bladder) can and does cause mechanical damage. Catheters can misshape cells, can adhere to and strip them away (denudation), and can leave the urethra in worse structural and functional condition after than before catheterization. Moreover, removing and/or otherwise damaging endothelial cells disrupts their physiological interactions with underlying smooth muscle cells and nerves. This can affect the contraction of the urethra, the streamlined flow of urine through it, and a number of other physiological and biochemical properties. Patients are usually not informed of these serious side effects before the physician inserts the catheter.

Additionally, no matter what surgical procedure is used to treat BPH or OAB, if it involves catheterization of the urethra, then it must also involve incising, puncturing, and/or otherwise damaging the urethra at the point of surgery. Remember, the prostate lies outside the urethra. Any attempts to cut, cauterize, irradiate, or pass laser beams into the prostate must first involve the wall of the urethra (or other tubular organ such as the rectum). So, in addition to the damage that intra-urethral devices do to the endothelium, damage is also done at the site of incision and cauterization (for example, the wall of the urethra, surrounding interstitial spaces, and the extracellular matrix). Before you agree to have one of these procedures, question the physician about the points I have just described. He or she should be able to give explanations that will satisfy your concerns. For example, you might ask about what effects intra-urethral scar tissue will have on the behavior of your urinary tract as you age further.

Treatment of Overactive Urinary Bladder in Women

Loss of control of the bladder is a taxing problem that is common in older women. In defining the overactive bladder and considering the complexity of symptoms, the International Continence Society (ICS) has highlighted the significant role of urgency. Urgency, an abnormal sensation, signifies impending or actual loss of control of the bladder and is accompanied by a fear of leakage. Urgency is important because it is thought to play a pivotal role in driving the other symptoms of urinary incontinence—that is, frequency and nocturia (getting up at night to urinate). Urgency is thought to reduce the time that voiding can be deferred, thereby increasing the frequency of urination and reducing the volumes eliminated (similar to BPH in men).

Overactive bladder syndrome is defined by the ICS as urgency with or without urge incontinence (the inability to control leaking and/or emptying of the bladder when urged). Aging women's reduced ability to store urine in the bladder has impacts on all aspects of life, including familial, societal, psychological, and professional ones. Incontinence in some women has been attributed to overactivity of the detrusor muscle, the smooth muscle in the bladder wall (detrusor overactivity, or DO). To rule out DO as a cause of incontinence, one group of investigators studied women ages twenty to eighty-five years. They divided their subjects by age and then into subgroups with and without DO. They reported that regardless of the presence or absence of DO, the lower urinary tract of women lost function with age.

Other investigators believe that similar loss of function occurs in men. In women specifically, studies have found that the strength of contractility of the bladder wall, sensitivity of the bladder to filling, and volitional control over urethral sphincters decline from young adulthood (ages twenty to thirty-nine) through early old age (ages sixty and older). Conversely, the capacity of the bladder to store urine and the frequency of urination during the daytime do not change with age in women. Of course, these last findings depend on one's degree of hydration. Anyone can intentionally become overhydrated or dehydrated. A woman who is overhydrated will urinate more frequently (and a woman who is dehydrated will urinate less often) during the waking hours than a woman who is normally hydrated. A friend who recently completed chemo- and radiation therapy for breast cancer told me that she had consulted other women who had undergone the therapy. The most frequent advice she got was to stay well hydrated. Two women told her to drink at least 100 ounces (about 3,000 mL) of water each day.

Since I have never been treated with chemo- or radiation therapy for breast cancer, I don't know how dehydrating those procedures can be or how they make one thirst. However, if my friend followed this advice, she and women like her must have been camping out in the restroom. If one adds to that 3,000 mL the water consumed from both indirect and intrinsic sources, my friend would always have been seriously overhydrated. Moreover, an aging woman with an overactive bladder would make even more trips to the bathroom and would be excreting larger volumes of more diluted urine on a nearly continuous basis. Needless to say, this would be unnecessary and even unhealthy.

Studies similar to those I have described above have been conducted to identify the effects of aging on the brain-bladder control system in women. This system refers specifically to the central regulation of the urination reflex in the brain, brainstem, and spinal cord. In these studies, women have been divided into two age groups, younger and older. As their bladders were experimentally filled with fluid, MRIs were taken of the brain regions thought to control urination. Images were collected as maximum volumes of the bladder were approached and during intentional incontinence (caused by pushing on the pelvic region or running cold water over the hand). The brain regions of greatest interest are the pons in the brainstem and the right insula and anterior cingulate of the cerebral hemispheres.

In subjects having no signs of bladder overactivity, increasing stretch of the bladder during filling led to increasing insular responses. With increasing age, insular responses became weaker. In younger subjects, the anterior cingulate region responded strongly at large volumes. Older women showed strong responses in the anterior cingulate even at small volumes, but more moderate responses at larger volumes. In subjects with an overactive bladder, activity in the micturition center of the pons did not increase with distension of the bladder. Such investigations reveal that among normal control subjects, increasing age leads to decreased responses in brain regions involved in control of the bladder.

Compounds that inhibit the actions of acetylcholine (anticholinergic and antimuscarinic compounds) are the mainstay of pharmacotherapy for the overactive female bladder. Acetylcholine is a naturally occurring neurotransmitter released by nerves that innervate the bladder, sphincters, and ureters. These drugs produce their effects by preventing acetylcholine from binding to its receptors. Recent experiments suggest that acetylcholine can also be released from nonneuronal sources by stretching the urothelium (endothelial cells lining the urethra). Also, there is increasing evidence that the neurotransmitter might act on receptors in nerve plexuses of the urethra, thereby influencing the afferent nervous system and detrusor contraction.

In one study, subjects kept a three-day micturition diary before their first office visit and before subsequent monthly visits (at weeks four, eight, and twelve). Subjects also underwent a baseline assessment. Data on urgency, incontinence, frequency of urination, episodes of nocturia, and volume of urine voided were collected using these three-day diaries. The time of rising from and going to bed were also recorded. Results for urgency, incontinence, frequency of micturition, volume of urine voided, and nocturia suggested that doses of 5–10 milligrams of anticholinergics (such as solifenacin) were effective in reducing the symptoms of the overactive bladder in women. When compared with the use of a placebo, treatment with solifenacin resulted in significant improvement in all the symptoms measured. In addition, at least one-third of the patients treated with solifenacin experienced normalization of the frequency of urination to eight or fewer episodes per day. Results also showed that solifenacin improved the patients' perception of the condition of their bladders.

Other investigators have studied the efficacy and safety of repeated injections of botulinum toxin-A (BTX-A, or Botox) in treating overactive bladder that did not respond to anticholinergics. In one study, patients received 200 units of Botox initially, with subsequent injections of 100–300 units administered via catheterization of the bladder. Efficacy was estimated using diaries of voiding, quality of life, and questions from standardized international surveys. Urodynamic data (pressure and volume in the bladder and rate of urine flow) were obtained before and for three months after the first three injections of the drug.

Significant improvements in the symptoms of overactive bladder and in the quality of life were observed after each injection when compared with baseline. Elasticity or compliance of the bladder also increased during the storage phase of urine production. Unfortunately, when researchers compared bladder function three months after the first and last injections of Botox, they found no significant differences. That is to say, there were no long-term benefits of this treatment (if six months can even be considered long term). The most common problems reported with the use of this drug were difficulty in emptying the bladder and urinary tract infections.

In another study, a subgroup analysis was undertaken of data from women eighteen years and older whose problems with overactive bladder had lasted longer than six months. Subjects were eligible for inclusion in this study if they reported urinary urgency at least once each three days; frequency of urination equal to or greater than ten times in any twenty-four-hour period; and urinary incontinence, with an average of more than one episode per day. Their information was recorded in diaries kept for three days following a seven-day washout period, during which no medication for the problems was permitted. This investigation found that trospium chloride, as an extended-release capsule, was well tolerated by women and was effective in significantly attenuating symptoms of the disorder. No long-term results were reported.

The above results should be useful to women seeking drug-related therapy for overactive bladder. These and related results provide a reference with which to compare current or future drug treatments proposed by a urologist. In approaches to treatments such as these, a woman should

carefully weigh the benefits (such as drug-related short-term improvements) and the risks (for example, difficulty urinating and infections)
before deciding whether or not to try drug therapy.

Sensation and Motor Control of the Bladder

Normal sensations from filling of the bladder and desire to void are
detected in the brain. This allows the central nervous system to exert physiological control. For example, in some mammals the hypothalamus has
direct access to the micturition center of the pons in the brainstem. Also,
junctions of the temporal and parietal lobes of the human cerebral cortex
are adjacent to regions of the brain that are activated by increasing volumes in the bladder. The general effect of increasing age on these regions
is a decrease in brain response. This might be due to a decrease in the
mass of neurons. It could also be influenced by a decrease in the activity of
sensory afferent nerves leaving the bladder, which would reduce sensory
feedback from the bladder. That would make control of the bladder more
difficult and perhaps lead to the development of urge incontinence in
older people.

The generally positive correlation of brain responses with age indicates that urge incontinence has different characteristics in older and
younger people. Younger individuals show reduced responses at smaller
volumes, as if they were neglecting information from the bladder. Among
normal control subjects, increased responsiveness in the right-insular
region of the brain at large volumes in the bladder (that is, having a strong
desire to void) and aging-related reduced responsiveness suggest that this
region of the brain helps monitor bladder function. For subjects who have
urge incontinence, however, it is questionable whether—as is commonly
believed—sensations and afferent signals are abnormally strong. At least
in younger people, their responses are weaker than normal at smaller volumes in the bladder. In these people even when the sensation to urinate is
strong, it might be different from the normally strong desire to do so.

Other studies show that the distinguishing characteristic of cases with
urge incontinence is strong activation of the anterior cingulate gyrus. The
anterior cingulate gyrus belongs to the limbic (emotional) nervous system,
and thus its activation suggests the involvement of emotion. This is to be

expected for the unusual sensations of urgency that are characteristic in women with OAB and men with BPH. Thus, a strong response of the anterior cingulate gyrus to filling of the bladder might be the functional MRI sign of urgency. It is unlikely, however, to be the cause of urgency. Simultaneous responses elsewhere in the brain (such as in the left parietal cortex) suggest that when loss of volitional control of the bladder is feared, activation of the anterior cingulate gyrus becomes part of the recruitment of alternative nerve pathways.

Anatomically, the anterior cingulate gyrus is a large region with several presumed functions. The region that is activated in response to filling of the bladder is also concerned with regulation of heart rate and other cardiovascular variables that respond to emotional stimuli. Possibly, in response to urgency, it might exert similar motor regulation of bladder behavior via brainstem nuclei. The nerve pathway must be indirect, however, since the anterior cingulate gyrus has no direct connection to the micturition center of the pons. More likely, activation of the anterior cingulate gyrus seems to be an emotional response to threatened loss of control of the bladder. Therefore, one might expect that its action on the micturition center of the pons should be inhibitory. The experimental evidence supports this notion.

In older subjects when there is no obstruction of the detrusor, activation of the anterior cingulate gyrus is strongest at small volumes, which implies adequate inhibition of the micturition center in the pons. At large volumes, however, inhibition might fail when obstruction of the detrusor is present. If so, the response of the anterior cingulate gyrus becomes correspondingly weaker. An alternative hypothesis concerning this paradoxical behavior in the elderly might be that age-related changes in afferent signals can provoke strong brain responses even at smaller volumes. In Parkinson's disease, perhaps for similar reasons, the micturition center of the pons is apparently not active during detrusor obstruction.

Among normal subjects, brain responses to filling of the bladder decline with increasing age. This is particularly true in the right insula, where normal sensations from the bladder are monitored. In subjects with urge incontinence, brain responses to filling of the bladder differ greatly between young and old. In both age groups, the responses are different from those in healthy people, even when no obstruction of the detrusor is present. Strong activation of selective regions of the brain is characteristic of all people with urge incontinence. It is probably a sign of the abnormal sensation of urgency. However, it might indicate recruitment of alternative pathways in the face of fear of leakage. In any case, it seems to have an inhibitory effect on the micturition center of the brainstem. The underlying cerebral cause of urge incontinence and detrusor obstruction remains uncertain, but it might be related to dysfunction of the prefrontal cortex.

Reflux of bladder contents into the ureters and kidneys (vesicoureteral reflux) can occur with age and disease. Such reflux of urine can affect both the structure and function of the kidneys. For example, before urine is passed into the ureters en route to the bladder, it is temporarily stored in the renal calyses (singular: calyx) and pelvis. Reflux can affect the volume, shape, and function of these regions of the inner kidney. Corresponding changes in the thickness and function of the overlying renal medulla and cortex also occur. At its worst, pressure in the pelvis, calyses, and upstream nephrons can increase to dangerous levels, sometimes shutting down renal function. This would be akin to uncorrected ureteral obstruction by a kidney stone or stones.

After several hours of ureteral obstruction by a kidney stone, in the young or aged, enough fluid can back up to cause hydronephrosis (excess water or ultrafiltrate in the nephrons). Also, dilation of the renal pelvis and calyses can develop over a period of hours to several days. Patients with this condition complain of severe pain (renal colic) resulting from distension of urinary structures and activation of pain receptors in the ureters. The pain of ureteral kidney stones, which is associated with violent peristaltic contractions upstream of the obstruction, is among the most severe encountered in clinical practice. If the obstruction is not removed, it can cause marked renal dysfunction and even acute renal failure (for example, the glomeruli can stop filtering plasma). Acute renal failure can lead to death.

When treating renal disease in the aging, resistance of different strains of bacteria to medication can also be a problem. For example, one seventy-five-year-old woman was discharged from the hospital after being treated for a urinary tract infection caused by a bacterium, *Pseudomonas aeruginosa*. She was subsequently readmitted for a painful left knee after an uncomplicated fall. At that time, she was clinically stable except for mild hypotension (94/47 millimeters of mercury) and a moderate effusion in the left knee. Aspirated fluid from the knee joint appeared grossly purulent, and in a culture of the fluid, bacteria grew that were sensitive to several antibiotics. Although the patient was treated with intravenous antibiotics, on the sixth day of hospitalization she developed anuria (lack of the production or flow of urine) and delirium. A renal ultrasound did not identify an obstructive problem in the urinary tract, but on the seventh day her renal failure worsened and she died. An autopsy confirmed septic arthritis due to *Pseudomonas aeruginosa*.

Pseudomonas aeruginosa is a rare cause of septic arthritis in the older patient. In contrast, it is well documented in children and young adults who are hospitalized with septic arthritis following traumatic wounds. The elderly woman referred to above had risk factors including poorly controlled diabetes and an amputation below the knee for vascular insufficiency. Her physicians reasoned that although her blood and urine cultures were negative on admission, the joint infection followed the spread of the organism from her previous urinary tract infection to the blood. It is probable that her knee trauma caused damage to the microvasculature that permitted the pathogen to enter the joint.

Treatment of aging men and women with androgen supplements is increasing. Androgens are a class of male reproductive hormones that include testosterone. The supplements are given to postmenopausal women mainly to improve their libido and to prevent and treat osteoporosis. They are given to aging men to improve muscle mass, bone strength, libido, erectile dysfunction, and overall quality of life. Sometimes they are given in combination with phosphodiesterase-5 inhibitors such as Cialis, Levitra, and Viagra. Increased use of androgen supplements in aging individuals has occurred despite the fact that there have been no rigorous clinical trials to examine their effects on the risk of cardiovascular, renal, and other diseases. This is problematic because studies in humans and animals have suggested that androgens can increase blood pressure and compromise renal function. Furthermore, kidneys contain the enzymes necessary to produce androgens de novo. Because of their gender, aging men are already at greater risk for cardiovascular and renal disease than women, despite the fact that plasma testosterone levels decrease significantly with age and chronic disease.

Some investigators hypothesize that this decrease is a protective mechanism against an even greater incidence of cardiovascular and renal disease and poorer outcomes. If that is true, then androgen supplements in aging men could negate this natural protective mechanism. Other researchers hypothesize that androgens augment the reabsorption of sodium and water in the proximal tubule, causing a reduction in their delivery to sensitive, regulatory vascular or tubular structures in the downstream nephron. This could lead to a feedback-induced increase in glomerular capillary pressure and filtration of sodium and water to compensate. Such increases could be harmful to the physiological homeostasis of water and sodium balance in the elderly. The interested reader who desires more information should research the topic "tubuloglomerular feedback" and the integration of salt and water homeostasis.

Menopause increases a woman's risk for cardiovascular and renal diseases. However, because of their gender, women are somewhat better protected than men against those diseases. Thus, androgen supplements might increase the risk of renal injury and cardiovascular disease in postmenopausal women to levels similar to those in men. It is also possible that circulating concentrations of androgens might increase naturally with age in some women and could further escalate risk factors for disease. As with estradiol-progesterone replacement therapy in postmenopausal women, it is likely that some healthy, active, aging men and women would not have adverse cardiovascular consequences with androgen supplements. It is equally conceivable that such men and women might not even need hormone replacement. However, in view of the increasing experimental evidence that supplemental androgens promote cardiovascular and renal disease, even when the circulating plasma concentrations are decreased, aging men and women who have the predisposition to cardiovascular and renal diseases should take androgen supplements only with caution.

7

The Aging Gastrointestinal System

While writing this chapter, I interviewed a sixty-four-year-old woman. She had experienced abdominal bloating, gas, and discomfort for most of her adult life. Her bowel movements were irregular, and her stools were compacted and of small volumes. She had seen multiple physicians including gastroenterologists as well as chiropractors, and other practitioners of alternative medicine, and none had been able to provide lasting help. After much reading and studying, at age sixty-two she decided to change her diet methodically and incrementally. She began replacing products containing refined flours and sugars with generous quantities of home-made salads, vegetables, and fruits. She basically eliminated sweets such as cakes, candies, pastries, and pies, and she ate meat sparingly and fish or chicken once or twice a week.

This transition in diet took her eighteen to twenty-four months to complete. In the process, her gastrointestinal symptoms (including bloating) disappeared, her bowel movements became more regular, and her stools were softer. Moreover, the inflammation of her joints and kinked hips, which had also been long-standing problems, disappeared. The range of motion in her shoulders, arms, back, and knees all improved markedly. Her conclusion: a diet that was consistently lacking in sufficient quantities and qualities of fiber, greens, colors, vitamins, and minerals had been the cause of her gastrointestinal and joint problems. Her self-diagnosis and disciplined nutrition gave her a new lease on life. She was not a vindictive woman, but she must have wanted to revisit those physicians to bill them for wasting her time and taking her money.

The Aging Oral Cavity

The gastrointestinal tract (GIT)—also known by such names as the gastrointestinal system, enterohepatic system, and alimentary tract—in humans and other mammals begins at the mouth (the oral end, or cephalad terminus) and ends at the anus (the aboral end, or caudal terminus). From a secretory perspective, both the nasal passages and the sinuses might be considered part of the GIT. Their secretory products often end up in the stomach and small intestine, where they are broken down, absorbed, and recirculated. However, it is more common to associate the nasal passages and sinuses with the respiratory system, where they play roles in filtering, humidifying, and regulating the temperature of inspired air. The effects of aging on the gastrointestinal system are seen in all tissues from the teeth and tonsils to the terminal anal sphincters.

Poor oral health is often associated with low economic status (for example, through the lack or loss of dental insurance), and reduced economic status can be associated with unhealthy aging. Having physical disabilities that limit one's capacity to take care of one's teeth and oral cavity (such as the lack of range of motion with arthritis and/or impairment of the motor nerves that control the arms and hands) can also lead to poor oral health. With aging, the appearance, function, and structure of the teeth and gums can change. Yellowing or darkening can be caused by changes in the composition and thickness of the enamel and its underlying dentin. Abrasion and the loss of teeth can contribute to the worsening appearance and health of the oral cavity. Moreover, declining blood flow occurs with age, and this means a loss of vascularity to the teeth and gums. Because the corresponding nerves are not being nourished as they were in our youth and younger adulthood, our teeth and gums lose sensitivity as we age. This can reduce responsiveness to trauma and diseases of the mouth.

Cementum (the substance that covers the surfaces of the roots of our teeth) begins to thicken with age, with the total amount nearly tripling between childhood and age seventy-five. Because cementum, like all tissues of the body, is composed primarily of hydrocarbon molecules, it can react with sugars (glycation, glycoxidation) and acids (acidification) in the things we eat and drink. Cementum also reacts with other chemicals we inhale or ingest, such as chewing tobacco, cigarette smoke, nicotine, methyl xanthines in coffee and tea, and alcohol. Individually and collectively, these agents can have a dehydrating and dessicating influence on the oral cavity and thereby counteract the secretions of salivary and other glands that are designed to keep the mouth moist and healthy.

Age-related changes in the oral mucosa and dietary, hormonal, and humoral deficiencies cause dehydration and thinning of the epithelial structures of the oral and nasal cavities as well as the larynx, pharynx, and downstream tissues of the GIT. Moreover, the width and content of muscle fibers of the periodontal ligament, part of the superstructure of the periodontium, decrease with age. This can have pronounced effects on the alignment and health of the teeth and gum lines. Deterioration and recession of the gingiva with age can lead to exposure of the cementum, thus contributing to caries and gingivitis. Although gingivitis is more common in the elderly population, age alone is not a risk factor for this disease or for periodontitis. Both can be reversed with good oral hygiene despite the patient's age.

With or without aging, periodontitis occurs when edema and inflammation of the gingiva cause the periodontal ligament to detach from the cementum and tooth structure. This eventually leads to increased depth of the gingival pocket and to loosening and loss of the teeth. Many older people are subject to periodontal detachment and loss of teeth because of poor oral hygiene and recession of the gingiva. In such people periodontitis has been associated with cardiovascular disease, loss of control of diabetes, reduced healing of wounds and injuries, and aspiration of the pathogens that cause pneumonia. This is particularly true in institutionalized and neglected elderly people.

To reduce these risks, prevention of periodontal disease is best achieved by brushing and flossing your teeth daily, visiting the dental hygienist and dentist at least semi-annually, and taking other preventive measures such as rinsing or gargling with mouthwash or hydrogen peroxide. Oral antibiotics such as doxycycline have been used as adjuncts for the treatment of older patients who are institutionalized. Coupled with regular dental care, these interventions can reduce the need to have teeth extracted. Among other things, plaque on teeth and gums is a biofilm of gram negative bacteria and the endotoxins they produce. These can concentrate at the gingival margins, leading to edema and inflammation and easily bleeding gums. Release of endotoxins into injured tissues compounds the problems associated with edema and inflammation. Moreover, oral endotoxins can be aspirated, swallowed, or otherwise absorbed into the pulmonary and systemic circulations, leading to more serious consequences such as endotoxemia, hospitalization, and even death.

The Aging Esophagus

The esophagus originates at the upper esophageal sphincter. That sphincter relaxes to permit the entry of food when one swallows. The swallowing reflex is activated when we voluntarily elevate the tongue and push a bolus of chewed food to the back of the mouth. The reflex is operated from the brainstem. Among other things, the reflex moves the epiglottis into the closed position to prevent food from entering the trachea. Swallowing also relaxes the upper esophageal sphincter momentarily, then closes it after the bolus of food has passed. A wave of muscle contraction pushes the bolus of food downstream into the esophagus. Subsequently, nerve activity and local distension of the esophagus open, then close, the lower esophageal sphincter and relax the stomach to prepare it for the arrival of a new meal.

Other physiological details of the swallowing reflex are beyond the scope of this book, but it is one of the most complicated and precisely coordinated reflexes known. Obviously it affects both the gastrointestinal and respiratory systems as well as others like the central and peripheral nervous systems. Aging not only affects the swallowing reflex overall, but it also influences each component of the reflex. Overall, the age-related changes in esophageal physiology seem to be mild or minimal in the healthy older person. However, difficulty swallowing (dysphagia) and gastroesophageal reflux disease (GERD) occur extremely frequently in elderly patients.

In the Western world, 10–20 percent of the population is affected by GERD. Many if not most of the cases are associated with strokes. GERD is usually caused by aphysiological relaxation of the lower esophageal sphincter, which allows reflux of stomach contents into the esophagus. It can also be caused by a hiatal hernia, which is a protrusion of the junction of the esophagus and stomach across the diaphragm and into the thoracic cavity, caused by weakening of the diaphragm or by congenital anomalies. These changes can be temporary or permanent. Altering eating and drinking behavior is usually recommended to help correct GERD, but medications such as proton pump inhibitors (which impair the release of acid by the stomach), histamine receptor blockers, and antacids are frequently prescribed. Surgery might be an option in those cases that do not improve with medications and changes in diet.

Swallowing disorders and GERD are often undiagnosed and therefore untreated in geriatric patients. In many cases, the optimal mode of treatment in the elderly has not been established or options for treatment are insufficient. Moreover, the incidence of adenocarcinoma of the esophagus and upper portions of the stomach associated with long-standing GERD and Barrett's esophagus has increased rapidly over the past two to three decades. In addition, a gradual decrease of pressure inside the upper esophageal sphincter occurs with age, causing a delay in relaxation after swallowing. Pressures associated with pharyngeal contraction and the velocity of esophageal peristaltic contractions also notably increase with age. These changes are attributed to increased resistance of transitional muscle at the upper esophageal sphincter, as compliance decreases during aging. Transitional muscle is a region where skeletal muscle is linearly replaced by visceral smooth muscle.

The sensory threshold for initiation of the swallowing reflex might also increase with age, and there is a significantly increased occurrence of near-simultaneous contractions, as well as failure of contractions after swallowing, in the distal esophagus. Also, radiographic and other imaging data have demonstrated more frequently occurring abnormalities of esophageal transit time in elderly people. Transit time is the period it takes a bolus of food to pass from the upper esophageal sphincter into the stomach. Finally, there have been conflicting results for the effects of aging on the function of the lower esophageal sphincter, the pressures it generates during swallowing, and the passage of peristaltic contractions through it.

Ten percent of people over age fifty report problems swallowing, although the majority of these people do not see their physicians for the condition. In the elderly, difficulties with swallowing are correlated with morbidity and even mortality. For example, institutionalized patients with dysphagia have significantly higher six-month mortality rates than those without the disorder. Increased morbidity and mortality have also been found in patients whose swallowing difficulties originate in the oral cavity and/or the pharynx, and whose difficulties are associated with accidental intake of food into the trachea (aspiration). Difficulty with swallowing can result from a variety of defects affecting the oral cavity, pharynx, or esophagus. Taking clinical histories, observing patients swallowing, and examining them with endoscopes and reviewing radiographic images allow clinicians to differentiate between oral and esophageal causes of dysphagia, and to distinguish structural or functional causes of the disease. This body of investigation reveals that the swallowing problems of most elderly people is pathophysiological—that is, they have functional dysphagia.

Even in the nondiseased elderly, video fluoroscopy reveals abnormalities in the passage of food from the mouth to the esophagus in up to 63 percent of those examined. It therefore seems likely that swallowing disorders are underdiagnosed and undertreated in the elderly. Swallowing disorders are most commonly seen in patients with cognitive or neurological deficits. A substantial number of institutionalized elderly patients have permanently impaired swallowing, necessitating surgical interventions to facilitate feeding. These surgical procedures include gastrostomy, jejunostomy, and the permanent installation of shunts or bypasses. Surgical sectioning of muscle can be used to treat some patients with documented obstruction caused by the offending muscles, and injections of Botox have offered a therapeutic alternative to surgery in others.

Primary disorders of motility of the esophagus are easily identified in older people with functional esophageal disease. These disorders include the failure of sphincters to relax and generalized esophageal spasm. Elderly patients with cognitive or neurological disorders respond poorly to medical treatment of functional esophageal disease. However, they respond well to pneumatic dilation. In this procedure, a balloon is temporarily inserted and placed at the levels of the problematic sphincters or in the main body of the esophagus. It is then inflated for a few minutes and subsequently deflated. This seems to correct the muscle problem, at least temporarily.

Failure of these patients to respond to therapy may be a result of the age-related deterioration of groups of nerve cell bodies (ganglia) that help control the contraction and relaxation of smooth muscle in the GIT. Injections of Botox into the lower esophageal sphincter can relieve symptoms of functional esophageal disease in older patients. Because it is less invasive than surgical techniques such as the installation of a feeding shunt, Botox injection might become the treatment of choice in the elderly. Other diseases such as diabetes, Parkinson's disease, hiatal hernia, and neuropathy in older people also have an increased incidence that is associated with impaired esophageal motility.

The Aging Stomach

One guiding principle in the consumption of food is that we should eat to live and not live to eat. Humans and other animals can live for long periods of time on very little food. A seventy-kilogram adult has sufficient carbohydrates in the circulation and liver to sustain him or her for one or two days. Moreover, stored protein can keep a person healthy and alive for an additional ten or twelve days. Finally, the amount of fat stored in fat cells, liver, and muscle can keep the same person alive for forty or fifty days. Collectively, these three reserves of readily available fuel energy can sustain life, without consumption of food and in the absence of disease, for sixty to seventy days. Of course, in today's overweight and obese societies, the average adult weighs more than seventy kilograms. Arguably, fat stores in many of the obese could sustain life for more than sixty or seventy days. However, as a word of warning, prolonged underfeeding and excessive fasting can be as dangerous as overeating.

As we approach seventy years of age, humans tend to lose weight. This appears to be due to the physiological anorexia of aging (loss of appetite), sarcopenia, and to a lesser extent the loss of fat mass. The causes of physiological anorexia of aging include changes in taste and smell, reduced body mass and caloric demand, and a decrease in adaptive relaxation of the stomach, which leads to hastened filling of the antrum and thus to early satiation (feeling full and satisfied). However, don't let this lull you into a false sense of security, the attitude that I can overeat before age seventy because I will lose weight after that point. With age it might also be progressively more difficult to shed extra pounds.

The human stomach can be divided into at least three components: the fundus (the proximal portion, near the junction of the lower esophageal sphincter), the corpus (or body, the majority of the stomach mass with its greater and lesser curvatures), and the antrum (the distal portion, which joins with the duodenum or first segment of the small intestine). The junction between the antrum and the duodenum is the pylorus. One of its anatomical features is the pyloric sphincter, the muscle collar that helps regulate the rate of emptying of a full stomach. Near the border of the fundus and corpus is an area of cells called the cardia. These cells behave like a pacemaker for the stomach. They initiate waves of peristaltic contractions that influence the storage and emptying of chyme, the mixture of semidigested food created in the stomach during ingestion of a meal.

Unlike the esophagus, the proximal third of which is composed of striated skeletal muscle, the stomach is composed solely of visceral smooth muscle. Three layers of visceral smooth muscle characterize all structures of the GIT. These include an outer longitudinal layer whose cells are arranged in parallel to the long axis of the organ, an inner circular layer with cells arranged perpendicular to the long axis, and a muscularis mucosae layer found beneath the circular layer and overlying the luminal mucosa (see a good medical dictionary or textbook on physiology for details and explanations; alternatively search googleimages.com).

Physiologically, the gastrointestinal system is characterized by its four most important functions, arranged alphabetically here: absorption, digestion, motility (muscle movements such as contraction and relaxation), and secretion. All of these functions are affected by our lifestyles and daily routines, including the liquids, solids, and medications we consume. The functions are also affected by the activities we engage in. For example, it is estimated that more than 30 million people worldwide consume nonsteroidal anti-inflammatory drugs (NSAIDS) such as ibuprofen. About half of these are elderly people, who take NSAIDS to relieve pain and reduce inflammation. Most of these users are unaware of the dangerous side effects the NSAIDS have, including erosion of the mucosal linings of the GIT and creation of bleeding ulcers and related conditions.

Numerous experiments and the collection of epidemiological information in humans have shown that the use of NSAIDs is associated with gastropathy (combined disease of the GIT), and that NSAID-induced gastropathy and its life-threatening complications occur primarily in the elderly. Overall, the use of NSAIDs increases by a factor of two to four the risk of peptic ulcers and death, as well as associated complications such as perforation and hemorrhage of the wall of the GIT. In the United States alone, medical costs attributable to NSAID-related gastrointestinal disorders exceed four billion dollars annually. Increased use of NSAIDs among the elderly is an obvious risk factor for these conditions, and aging increases the likelihood of people taking NSAIDs and developing complications from such use.

One of the first lines of defense against the damaging effects of gastric and peptic acids, as well as noxious substances ingested in the foods and drinks we consume, is a gelatinous, alkaline layer of mucus and bicarbonate ions that is secreted by the stomach, duodenum, and pancreas. This material coats the surface of the gastrointestinal mucosa and protects it from corrosive damage potentially caused by gastric acids. Advancing age is associated with a significant thinning of this protective mucosal barrier. There is also a decrease in fluid secretions, including bicarbonate ions and other buffers that come from cells other than those producing acids and pepsin. Conversely, there are no apparent age-related changes in the release of secretions by parietal cells, including those in the gastric pits that produce pepsin and gastric or hydrochloric acid.

The above findings are in agreement with data from studies in the rat, showing that aging is associated with significantly lower pH in the gastric lumen and release of bicarbonate ions in the stomach. Aging also attenuates the prostaglandin-mediated increases in the secretion of gastric bicarbonate in rats. Other experiments in rodents have shown that the duodenal bicarbonate response to injection of acid either in the stomach or duodenum declines progressively with age.

Ghrelin, a recently discovered hormone secreted by the stomach, stimulates eating, promotes the release of growth hormone, and inhibits the production of pro-inflammatory cytokines. Ghrelin also reverses age-related shrinkage of the thymus gland. Investigators have found that chronic restriction of food in aging mice not only results in loss of body weight but also leads to a significant increase in the size of the stomach. The increase is due largely to growth of the fundus and enlargement of the antrum. Microscopic and tissue analysis of serial segments of the stomach reveal that the growth is seen at all cellular levels of the aged animals. These same investigators reported that chronic restriction of food during aging significantly increases circulating concentrations of ghrelin and reverses age-related loss of its receptors in the pituitary gland. Such findings suggest that enlargement of the mouse stomach induced by the deprivation of food could be helpful to survival during periods of starvation.

Many healthy older men and women of normal weight decrease their intake of foods and calories below their expenditure of energy and thus lose weight. This loss of weight is associated with reductions in both the mass of muscle and fat, as well as with frailty, functional impairment, and mortality. Men and women after age seventy who lose weight are more likely to develop pressure ulcers, to fall and fracture their hips, and to become cognitively impaired. Their quality of life also decreases. Overall, the loss of weight generally leads to poor outcomes in older people. Thus, one of the conundrums of aging is that although restrictions of diet might prolong life, loss of weight in older men and women shortens life. In older humans it now appears that depression is the most common cause of the physiological anorexia that leads to the loss of weight.

Physical activity also declines over the life span and is associated with physiological anorexia. Physiological anorexia is inadequate to prevent obesity in many young and middle-aged men and women, but in older men and women it can outpace the reduction of physical activity, thereby leading to loss of weight and sarcopenia. In general, there are minimal changes in the extraction of energy from carbohydrates, fats, and proteins with aging. If aging-induced physiological anorexia is to be eliminated or at least attenuated, lifelong physical activity, including a focus on weight lifting and resistance exercises, appears to be essential. More detailed studies on the role of the noncompliant fundus of the stomach in the pathogenesis of aging-induced anorexia will also be needed.

Although the predominant change in eating seen in older people is a decrease in the consumption of food, some investigators have suggested that the major change is a dysregulation of the intake of food (dysorexia). These investigators have found that, when compared to younger men and women, older adults who are overfed are less capable of decreasing their intake of food and returning to their previous weight. Similarly, older people who were underfed continued to eat less and failed to regain their lost weight. Additionally, with aging there is a small increase in the threshold for taste, which is amplified in people who smoke or take medications. Correspondingly, there is a decline in the ability to detect odors. Detection of the aromas of food preparation is a key element in the enjoyment of food.

My wife has perfected the art of seasonal baking and cooking. I hope to always enjoy being greeted at the front door by the aromas of freshly baked homemade bread, stew, and chili. These wonderful odors have embellished the atmosphere of our home for more than forty-five winters. Slices of hot, homemade wheat bread spread with butter and honey are the Cinnabons of my life. One of my saddest thoughts is that I will no longer have these after death. Oh, that I could be wrong! The aromas, sights, and sounds of food being prepared work collectively to prepare the entire gastrointestinal system for such delicious meals. Still, there is much controversy on the exact effects of alterations in taste and smell over the life span and how these influence our intake of food with age. Happily, about a decade ago it was shown that addition of the taste enhancer monosodium glutamate (MSG) to a single meal in a nursing home lead to a gain of weight among its residents. Perhaps there are other tastes and aromas waiting to be discovered that will also enhance the health and well-being of the elderly, whether or not they are institutionalized.

Because the threshold for detection of flavors increases with age, a higher concentration of any particular food must be eaten by an older person in order to recognize the product. Also, the number of acinar cells in the salivary glands declines with age. This means that the salivary products of those cells are also reduced, thereby impairing the gland's digestive effectiveness. In addition to digestive effects, adequate salivary function is important to prevent dryness of the mouth, to help humidify inspired air, to sustain vocalization, and to minimize or prevent dental disease. Therefore it is especially important for an elderly person to be vigilant about remaining hydrated. This is not achievable with water alone but depends also on the quality and quantity of the solutes contained in the water in the foods we eat. We must sustain a physiological balance between the depletion of these important life-giving elements and their replenishment.

The products of our meals reach the water compartments of our bodies, including the vascular space and blood. Our blood and plasma supply the salivary and other glands with raw materials that the glands use to make secretions.

Emptying the stomach following the ingestion of a meal is influenced by the composition of the meal. Liquid meals pass through the stomach more rapidly than solid meals do. Meals with high fat content are released more slowly from the stomach than those with little or no fat. Also, the greater the osmolarity of the meal, the longer it takes to leave the stomach. This means meals that are high in salt content will be emptied more slowly than those with less salt. Aging influences the rate of emptying of our stomachs. In one study it took about 125 minutes for half of an ingested meal to be emptied in elderly subjects, verses about 50 minutes in younger participants. In addition, both the baseline and stimulated release of gastric acid (stomach acid, peptic acid, and hydrochloric acid) have been shown to decrease in the elderly. This is problematic because stomach acid plays an important role in digesting proteins and detoxifying ingested pathogens.

Atrophy of the glands in the stomach that produce gastric acid also increases with age. Investigators have found that more than 40 percent of Bostonians age eighty and over have atrophic gastritis. *Helicobacter pylori* organisms, once thought to be harmless residents of the upper GIT, are now known to be associated with gastritis and cancer of the esophagus. In one study of subjects over age sixty, more than 80 percent of subjects with gastritis had blood-borne antibodies to *Helicobacter pylori* compared to less than 50 percent of those without gastritis. Gastritis in the elderly can be a factor not only in the impaired secretion of gastric acid but also in the impaired release of intrinsic factor (produced by the stomach, intrinsic factor is important in the absorption of vitamin B-12 by the ileum). Because of the malabsorption of vitamin B-12, impaired secretion of intrinsic factor can lead to pernicious anemia.

The Aging Small Intestine

The small intestine in humans extends from the stomach's pyloric sphincter to the junction of the ileum and the large intestine (the colon). The small intestine can be divided proximally to distally (from the oral to the aboral ends) into the duodenum, jejunum, and ileum. Each of these segments has unique structural and functional properties. As mentioned above, four general functions are served by the small intestine: absorption, digestion, motility, and secretion. Absorption means the transfer of products of digestion from the lumen of the gut into the systemic circulatory system. Digestion involves the breakdown of products of chyme, including: (1) the conversion of proteins and peptides into smaller amino acids; (2) the reduction of complex sugars such as glycogen and other macromolecular carbohydrates to simple sugars like fructose, glucose, and galactose; and (3) the transformation of complicated luminal lipids (fats) such as micelles into simpler units such as triglycerides, glycerol, and free fatty acids.

The products of digestion just described are taken up by mucosal epithelial cells that line the walls of the small intestine. Membranes of these cells contain integral proteins that serve as carriers, channels, enzymes, and pores. For example, some carriers recognize and bind only to acidic amino acids, others transport primarily basic amino acids, and still others carry only neutral amino acids. Glucose, a monosaccharide, is commonly transported in combination with sodium ions on the luminal side of the epithelial cell (SGLT1 transporter), but is transported by itself on the basal (interstitial, or circulation) side of the same cell (GLUT2 transporter). Triglycerides, the most common type of fat in our daily diets, are released from micelles at the mucosal border, reduced to glycerol and free fatty acids, and then transported into the epithelial cell. Once inside the epithelium, they are reconstituted into more complex units called chylomicrons. These are absorbed into the lymphatic circulation and from there are delivered to the systemic circulation.

Motility involves all movements of the GIT, including haustrations (localized indentations of the gut wall that do not move orally or aborally; these are seen predominantly in the colon or large intestine), peristalsis, propulsion, retropulsion, and segmentation. Generally speaking, peristalsis is the process by which chyme is moved in a net antegrade direction (from mouth to anus). The rate of peristalsis (several contractions per minute, varying between the fed and fasting states) is set by the cardia and tends to decrease segmentally from duodenum to colon (eight to ten contractions per minute in the proximal duodenum, decreasing to three to four per minute in the distal ileum). This arrangement ensures the net forward movement of chyme. Propulsion can be either antegrade or retrograde, and the stomach is a good example of this. In the full stomach, an antegrade wave of peristaltic contractions traveling from fundus to antrum can collide with a retrograde wave that originated in the antrum. The head-on collision of the two opposing waves causes additional mixing of the chyme, release of gases, and sometimes familiar sounds. The additional mixing ensures maximum exposure of the chyme (containing carbohydrates, fats, proteins, and secretory products) to corresponding enzymes and other digestive elements such as acid. This enhances the further processing of chyme once it enters the duodenum.

Gastrointestinal secretion begins in the mouth and ends in the colon. Secretion refers to the release of secretory products from glands such as the parotid and sublingual. Oral secretions are particularly helpful in initiating digestion of ingested carbohydrates. The primary example of such a secretion is alpha amylase, a product released from salivary glands that helps digest complex carbohydrates such as starches (for example, glycogen). Other secretions contain acids and enzymes (such as pepsinogen and lipase) needed to digest proteins and lipids. The above secretory functions, and others, are subject to change with aging.

Imagine that before eating you could liquefy and measure the volume of your meal. Imagine also that the volume is 500 mL. By the time a similar meal has been turned to chyme in the stomach and begins its journey through the small intestine, the addition of secretory products—including water—will have expanded the volume of 500 mL three to four times. Instead of the stomach having to accommodate the original meal of 500 mL, it might temporarily have to store 1,500–2,000 mL or more. Now think of the discomfort this might cause your abdominal cavity. So, as you prepare to ingest a meal (for example, a Thanksgiving dinner of 1,000 mL due to overeating), try to imagine the added volume of secretory products that will end up in the stomach and duodenum as a result of that meal. This might help you control your appetite and avoid the predictably uncomfortable postingestive state.

The intestinal brush border maximizes the surface area for digestion and absorption of a meal. The brush border is critical to the healthy function of the gastrointestinal tract. In animal experiments, the secretory glands of the intestinal brush border have been shown to decrease with age. Similar investigations have reported an age-dependent decrease in several key brush border enzymes, including lactase, maltase, and sucrase-isomaltase. Also, the surface area of the intestinal mucosa has been reported to decline in elderly humans when compared to younger subjects. Reduced surface area is an indirect indicator of the declining abundance of mucosal digestive and transport functions. Reduced brush borders and corresponding surface areas mean reduced digestion and transport of amino acids, simple sugars, and complex lipids.

Hydrogen gas in the exhaled air is one measure of incomplete digestion and absorption of carbohydrates. When elderly subjects (those ages sixty-five to eighty-nine years) were compared to younger subjects (ages twenty to sixty-four), investigators found that about a third of the older subjects exhaled excess hydrogen gas while none of the younger subjects did—a significant difference. This suggests malabsorption of carbohydrates in the elderly. However, in another study, the lactose-to-mannitol ratio in the plasma did not differ between young and old subjects, indicating that intestinal permeability to these sugars does not change significantly with age in humans.

It is reasonable to speculate that the complexity of absorption of lipids in the small intestine might make it susceptible to the effects of aging, and early work in humans has shown this to be the case. There appears to be reduced intestinal absorption of bile acids with age as well. However, it is not clear if this has a negative effect on the absorption of lipids in older people. Thus, the jury is still out on the effect of aging on the absorption of energy products by the small intestine. More work is needed.

The Aging Large Intestine

The human colon begins at the ileocecal valve and continues to the anus. When performing flexible colonoscopies, the gastroenterologist uses the ileocecal valve to help map the location of his endoscope. The human colon is composed of the cecum (the segment to which the appendix is attached) and the ascending, transverse, descending, and sigmoidal segments. In cancers of the gastrointestinal tract, the colon is the most commonly affected site. It is also the permanent residence of commensal bacteria—those that are symbiotic with the fauna and flora of the gut and contribute to GIT health.

Irritable bowel syndrome is one of the most common complaints among people of all ages. The most common symptoms are abdominal discomfort that is relieved by defecation, changes in the frequency of bowel movements, changes in the form of the stool (hard versus soft, small versus large volumes, and so on), the presence of mucus in the stool, and bloating or feelings of abdominal distension. The prevalence of irritable bowel syndrome is higher in women than in men, and in adults and the elderly compared to the young. The overall prevalence is 10–20 percent, and the condition accounts for 20–50 percent of all initial consultations with a gastroenterologist. Irritable bowel syndrome is frequently associated with constipation, diverticula of the colon, fibromyalgia, anxiety, and depression. Initial treatment is based on the modification of diet as well as the control of diarrhea with drugs and of constipation with laxatives, and the use of antidepressants. Organic disease such as a blockage of the intestinal lumen (for example, tumor at a sphincter) has to be ruled out, and this can usually be done with colonoscopies and magnetic resonance images (MRIs).

A number of years ago, my wife and I took a business and pleasure trip to Edinburgh, Scotland. The hotel had marvelous breakfast buffets. In addition to hot choices, there was a wide variety of fruits and nuts. We both tried adding almonds to hot oatmeal and found the result to be very enjoyable. After we returned, my wife began including almonds on her regular grocery shopping lists. Between the time of that trip and the time of this writing I have had several colonoscopies. The latest revealed a few polyps, and my gastroenterologist removed them. About that same time, I began having periodic bouts of what I would call irritable bowel syndrome. They arose without notice, usually in the late P.M. to early A.M. hours while I was in bed. The initial discomfort escalated into sustained, blunt, and diffuse pain in or near the descending or sigmoid colon. Each annoying and painful episode ended only after one or two uneventful trips to the bathroom, after moving my bowels, or spontaneously after fifteen to thirty minutes of lying awake in pain.

I experienced these gastrointestinal conditions once or twice per month for several years. In January 2013, and unrelated to irritable bowel syndrome, I shed several pounds and began a more serious review of my eating habits. Among other changes, I excluded almonds from my hot breakfast. After losing ten or twelve pounds and while reflecting on that experience, I realized that my episodes of irritable bowel syndrome had diminished or disappeared. I can't confirm my conclusions, but I attribute the cessation of these episodes to the removal of almonds from my diet. It is conceivable that the incompletely digested nuts were irritating the delicate mucosal lining of my colon, especially in or near the region of my more recent polypectomies. Perhaps the almonds even helped cause the polyps.

Irritable bowel syndrome is not necessarily the beginning of a spectrum of gastrointestinal ailments. Irregular bowel movements and constipation or diarrhea might play that role. Health professionals typically define constipation as having fewer than three bowel movements per week. However, the public defines constipation as any form of difficult defecation, including straining at stool, having hard stool, feeling of incomplete evacuation, and nonproductive urges to move one's bowels. In one study of 531 patients in a general practice, 50 percent gave a different definition of constipation than their physicians did. Because of the confusion, an international panel of experts proposed using a combination of subjective symptoms as criteria. Using them, investigators have reported that the prevalence of constipation increases with age, especially in people over sixty-five years.

Constipation disproportionately affects the elderly, with a prevalence of 50 percent in those living at home or with loved ones and 74 percent in residents of nursing homes. Moreover, aging women are two to three times more likely to report constipation than aging men are. Some of the known causes of constipation include loss of mobility, medications, underlying diseases, impaired anorectal sensation, ignoring the urge to defecate, and irritable bowel syndrome. It is noteworthy that elderly subjects with advanced dementia who live in nursing homes, as well as those on opioids for end-of-life care, usually require individualized approaches for the treatment of constipation.

Chronic primary constipation is manifested by persistent reductions in the frequency of bowel movements that are accompanied by sensations of difficult and seemingly incomplete emptying. Chronic primary constipation is the most common functional disturbance encountered in older people, and it can be associated with either normal or reduced transit rates in the large intestine. Like all functional digestive disorders, chronic primary constipation is diagnosed by the process of elimination or exclusion. As mentioned above, one of the first steps is to rule out organic or structural disease such as tumors.

The most frequent cause of constipation is the delayed transit of fecal matter in the colon as a result of reduced intestinal motility. In older people reduced intestinal motility is most likely to be associated with chewing deficiencies, reduced secretion of gastric acid, deficiencies in the intake of water and insoluble fiber, and limited physical activity (including immobile lifestyles). A number of diseases are also associated with constipation: (1) endocrine and metabolic disorders such as diabetes and hypothyroidism; (2) myopathy; (3) neurologic diseases and disorders, including cerebral ischemia and stroke, multiple sclerosis, and Parkinson's disease; (4) psychiatric disturbances such as depression and anxiety; and (5) structural colorectal disease such as tumor-induced stenosis, hemorrhoids, and rectal prolapse.

Drug-related constipation is also important and can be caused by antacids, anticholinergics, antidepressants, antihistamines, antihypertensives, antimitotics (for example, cholchicine), and other chemotherapeutics, hypnotics, and opioids. Treatment of chronic constipation is based on ensuring adequate intake of water, a diet rich in fiber (35–40 grams per day is ideal), olive oil, physical activity, and laxatives. Wheat and wheat-based cereals, both hot and cold, are ideal laxatives and are healthy alternatives to over-the-counter drugs. The daily intake of fiber should be no less than 15–20 grams and preferably twice this amount, with the majority of the fiber being insoluble as opposed to soluble.

There is a growing trend for physicians and the lay public to diagnose or self-diagnose celiac disease. This is the notion that wheat and wheat-based products cause many of the food allergies that humans complain about. I don't know if celiac disease is real or imagined. I do know that wheat—along with corn and rice—is one of the super grains of the world. With the possible exception of rice, more people and animals are sustained on wheat and wheat-based food products than on any other grain. Moreover, rice is mainly eaten by people in the eastern hemisphere because it is one of the few grain crops that can survive the rainy conditions in much of the region and is less expensive there than other grains. Gram for gram, rice is not nearly as healthy for you as wheat is.

Despite the bad reputation that celiac disorders—as well as dieticians, physicians, and others—have given to wheat in recent decades, I believe that wheat-based products are still among the best dietary components for avoiding constipation and other diseases of the digestive tract. Wheat, especially noncommercial products such as properly prepared whole or cracked wheat kernels and finely ground whole wheat flour (for home-made bread and so forth), is among the best sources of insoluble dietary fiber that can be found. Such noncommercial products frequently contain as much as 12–15 grams of insoluble fiber per 100 grams of whole or cracked wheat. Wheat also has a relatively high protein content. Moreover, because of its low content of moisture, whole wheat can be stored indefinitely (particularly hard, red, winter varieties).

Equally important, natural whole wheat grains are much less expensive per unit weight than commercially available, over-the-counter anti-cathartics (for example, generic laxatives, Metamucil, and Fibercon). This means almost everyone can afford to buy, store, and process their own high-fiber, dietary wheat products. I strongly recommend considering this as a first option to improved health of the colon, even before seeing a physician and consuming more medications. Other foods with high-fiber contents include bran-based cold cereals (such as Grape-Nuts), lentils, beans, and filamentous vegetables. Finally, there is an inverse correlation between one's consumption of insoluble fiber and diseases of the colon, including constipation. Insoluble fiber, more than any other natural dietary macronutrient, increases the retention of intraluminal water in the colon. The greater the contents of insoluble fiber and intraluminal water in the colon, the lower the chances for constipation.

Laxatives include lubricants such as vegetable and mineral oil, liquid paraffin, docusate sodium, and hydrating agents (osmotics) like magnesium hydroxide, magnesium sulfate, magnesium citrate, and sodium biphosphate. Unfortunately, all these can also cause depletion of potassium, retention of sodium and water, and diarrhea. The so-called bulk laxatives (psyllium, agar, methyl-cellulose) have been replaced by the use of high-fiber diets. The stimulant laxatives (senna, bisacodyl, cascara) increase peristalsis in the colon and promote the secretion of water and electrolytes from the gut wall. They can cause cramps and cathartic colon, conditions that are characterized by loss of muscle tone with accompanying dilation of the colon and loss of haustra. Prolonged use of stimulant laxatives can lead to depletion of electrolytes. More recently cholchicine has been approved by the Food and Drug Administration to increase propulsive activity in the gut. It is also noteworthy that in some countries, including Italy, mineral waters with laxative effects are available. Sulfate and sodium sulfate waters are particularly useful in these cases.

Fecal incontinence is the accidental, involuntary passage of feces or gas. The prevalence of this disorder is 2–7 percent in the elderly population in general, and over 45 percent among the institutionalized. Fecal continence depends on rectal compliance, anorectal sensitivity, function of the external and internal anal sphincters, and normal neuromuscular activity in the floor of the pelvis. Alterations that accompany aging include decreased rectal elasticity, decreased tone of the external anal sphincter, and decreased resting pressures in the internal anal sphincter. People displaying the signs of incontinence might suspect lesions of the anus and operative nerves, hemorrhoids, fissures, rectoceles, previous surgery, and systemic diseases that might favor the condition (such as diabetes, cognitive deficits, and neurological disease). The management of fecal incontinence frequently includes teaching the patient how to care for him- or herself, eliminating local causes of the condition such as inflammation and hemorrhoids, and treating systemic diseases that are either causing or contributing to the condition.

In the elderly, age-related neurodegenerative changes in the enteric nervous system have also been noted. In one study, investigators found a 37 percent loss of enteric neurons in people more than sixty-five years of age when compared with those ages twenty to thirty-five years. Another study showed the age-related loss of neurons that express an enzyme marker of enteric neurons. These and related findings suggest an increase in inhibitory neurons in the aging colon and reductions in motility of the gut. Unfortunately, the significance of such findings is still unclear. They could suggest either a primary malfunction or an indirect effect of the chronic use of laxatives in constipated patients through the years. In fact, gut transit time and colonic motility are similar in healthy older and younger participants. In contrast, elderly people reporting chronic constipation have a total gut transit time of four to nine days (the norm is less than three days). In the least mobile residents of nursing homes, transit times are prolonged up to three weeks. One GIT-related goal in aging should be the maintenance of a near-normal transit time of three to four days. This is best achieved through diet and nutrition.

The Aging Pancreas

The human pancreas has both endocrine and exocrine functions. For example, as an exocrine organ, the pancreas releases bicarbonate ions (which buffers the small intestine and other dowstream organs from the effects of hydrochloric acid produced by the stomach) and pancreatic lipases (enzymes to digest dietary lipids). These exocrine functions are important to the digestive and absorptive functions of the duodenum and downstream segments of the gut. As an endocrine organ, the pancreas releases insulin, glucagon, and somatostatin. They are produced, respectively, by the beta, alpha, and delta cells of the islets of Langerhans. All three hormones are important in energy metabolism, growth, and development.

Somatostatin was first discovered in the hypothalamus, where it was found to inhibit the release of growth hormone from the pituitary. Growth hormone is also known as somatotropin—hence, the name of somatostatin. Somatostatin also inhibits the release of multiple other hormones, including gastrin, glucagon, insulin, thyroid-stimulating hormone, and vasoactive intestinal peptide. Stimuli for the release of glucagon are amino acids from ingested proteins. Glucagon's main target of action is the liver, where it regulates the metabolism of carbohydrates and lipids. Glucagon is particularly important in stimulating the breakdown of glycogen (hepatic glycogenolysis) and in creating new glucose from amino acids (gluconeogenesis, also in the liver). Glucagon's actions are not limited to the liver: it causes glycogenolysis in both cardiac and skeletal muscle, as well as lipolysis in fat tissue.

Insulin regulates the supply of body fuels. It does this during both fasting and feeding and uses the physiological processes of glycogenolysis, gluconeogenesis, and lipolysis. These processes take place in target organs such as the liver, skeletal muscle, and fat depots. Collectively, they regulate the circulating concentrations of glucose or blood sugar. It is important that plasma levels of glucose remain relatively constant, at 80–100 milligrams per deciliter, to avoid both hypo- and hyperglycemia (a deficit and excess of glucose, respectively). Of all the organs, the brain and central nervous system are most dependent on the constancy of blood glucose. If circulating concentrations of glucose decline below 35–55 milligrams per deciliter for even a brief period, confusion, coma, and seizures can occur. Conversely, severe hyperglycemia (glucose concentrations above several hundred milligrams per deciliter) can lead to osmotic diuresis, severe dehydration, electrolyte imbalance, hypotension, and vascular collapse.

In healthy young or old people, plasma concentrations of glucose remain within a remarkably narrow range. After an overnight fast, the concentrations are 70–90 milligrams per deciliter (or 70–90 milligrams percent—that is, 70–90 milligrams per 100 milliliters of plasma). These numbers are elevated 30 to 120 minutes after normal meals but usually do not rise above 150–200 milligrams per deciliter even after large meals. Modest increases in plasma glucose cause marked secretion of pancreatic insulin, and hence an increase in the circulating concentrations of insulin. Conversely, a decline in glucose of only 20 percent significantly lowers plasma insulin. The changes in glucose that accompany feeding and fasting are the main determinants of the secretion of insulin.

In diabetics, diagnosed or not, an oral or intravenous challenge with glucose evokes a smaller increase in the secretion of insulin and therefore is accompanied by higher circulating concentrations of glucose for a prolonged period. For these reasons, oral and intravenous glucose tolerance tests are the clinical gold standards for diagnosing type I diabetes. I have had glucose tolerance tests performed on me, and in an experimental physiology laboratory I use this test to teach students the physiology of glucose and insulin. In both cases, an oral glucose test was (is) used.

An intravenous injection of about 0.5 grams glucose per kilogram of body weight, or about thirty-five grams of glucose in a seventy-kilogram person, raises the plasma glucose more rapidly than if the same quantity of glucose is given orally. The rapid rise in glucose leads to a biphasic insulin response. In the first phase, circulating concentrations of insulin rise within several minutes of the glucose challenge, and the increase lasts only two to five minutes. A secondary rise in insulin can be detected within thirty to sixty minutes and lasts as long as circulating concentrations of glucose remain elevated. The insulin released during the first phase comes from secretory granules that had previously stored insulin. The second phase comes from newly synthesized as well as previously stored insulin. Another sign of diabetes is the loss of the first phase of secretion of insulin during an intravenous glucose tolerance test.

Pancreatic beta cells extract and metabolize circulating monosaccharides such as fructose, glucose, and galactose, each of which can induce the secretion of insulin. Other six-carbon sugars (hexoses) or monosaccharides such as 2-deoxyglucose can be transported into the beta cells but are not metabolized and do not stimulate the secretion of insulin. From experimental data such as these, we know that the release of insulin involves at least several steps. First, glucose enters the beta cell by a special protein carrier (GLUT2, or glucose transporter 2) and facilitated diffusion. Second, once inside the cell, glucose is metabolized by glycolysis to elevate the cellular concentrations of adenosine triphosphate (ATP), a high-energy phosphate compound that is required for the secretion of insulin. Third, changes in ATP and/or its ratio to other adenine nucleotides causes closure of a specific potassium channel in the membrane of the beta cell. Fourth, closure of the potassium channel confines potassium inside the cell, the cell accumulates a net positive electrical charge, and the membrane depolarizes. Fifth, that depolarization activates membrane-bound calcium channels, which open and admit extracellular calcium. Sixth, intracellular concentrations of calcium increase. And seven, this leads to release or secretion of insulin.

Both the incidence and the prevalence of type II diabetes increase with age. As of this writing, the disease affects 20–30 percent of the elderly population in the United States. Unfortunately, the underlying mechanism(s) behind the effects of aging on diabetes are still not clearly understood. It has been hypothesized that insulin resistance increases with age due to increased obesity, decreased lean muscle mass, changes in dietary habits, and reduced physical activity. Still, these factors alone do not account for age-related glucose intolerance, nor does aging itself seem to be the culprit. For example, in one study comparing two groups of men, those ages eighteen to thirty-six and those ages fifty-seven to eighty-two, the subjects underwent frequent measurement of plasma glucose and insulin during an intravenous glucose tolerance test. When compared to the younger men, the older ones showed a significant decrease in the rate of removal of glucose from the blood, despite elevated plasma insulin. These data imply that insulin sensitivity decreases with age. In a different study of young men (ages nineteen to thirty-six) and older men (ages forty-seven to seventy-three), the removal of glucose from the plasma was found to be dependent on the waist-to-hip ratio and not on age. Higher waist-to-hip ratios were associated with impaired glucose clearance. The latter findings suggest that the distribution of body fat rather than age alone leads to insulin resistance.

Another study revealed a 25 percent decline in the rate of insulin delivery between ages eighteen and eighty-five. That study, employing both men and women, controlled for body mass index, fasting plasma glucose, and insulin sensitivity. Results suggest that the function of beta cells declines with age. In another study of young adults (ages twenty-three to twenty-five) and older adults (ages sixty-four to sixty-six), defects in the function of beta cells in older people were observed only in those with pre-existing impaired glucose tolerance or type II diabetes. Relative to their younger counterparts, older people with normal concentrations of glucose had similar insulin responses to hyperglycemia. The results of this study suggest there is not necessarily an overall age-related decrease in function of beta cells, but that dysfunction might be observed only in the setting of impaired glucose tolerance or frank diabetes.

Such whole-body (macroscopic) studies are difficult to interpret because glucose intolerance can develop from a combination of factors, and controlling for all of them is impossible. Therefore, more recent experiments have focused on the effects of aging on the beta cell, specifically on insulin secretion, mass of beta cells, and the proliferation and regeneration of those cells. Results suggest that alterations in the oxidation of glucose, efflux of potassium, and intracellular concentrations of ionized free calcium can influence the aging beta cell. Intracellularly, oxidation of glucose elevates the production of ATP. Therefore, reductions in the rate of oxidation of glucose with aging would result in reduced secretion of insulin because of impaired synthesis of ATP. Aging might also affect the potassium and calcium channels that are involved in the secretion of insulin. Normally, elevated glucose concentrations induce beta cells to inhibit potassium efflux, resulting in increased calcium influx. The increase in intracellular calcium induces insulin secretion.

In a study of potassium channels that compared three-month-old and twenty-four-month-old rats, researchers observed a significant potassium efflux even after high glucose stimulation in older rats, indicating that the normal inhibition of the ATP-sensitive potassium channel is lost with age. The researchers suggested that this might be due to the reduced expression of a specific transcription factor named FoxM1. FoxM1 regulates genes that are involved in cell cycling and cell division and is highly expressed in proliferating cells. However, its expression declines in most aging cells, including human pancreatic beta cells. Interestingly, a study of pancreatic glands from twenty nondiabetic organ donors ages seven to sixty-six years showed a decline in the replication of beta cells with age. The decline was associated with the reduced expression of another pancreatic and duodenal transcription factor known to be important for the replication of beta cells. A similar investigation of more than a hundred pancreatic glands from obese, diabetic, and lean people ages sixty-one to eighty-three at autopsy showed low-frequency replication of beta cells.

Finally, an increased incidence of diabetes is observed with age, and there are many possible explanations for this. One explanation is that the beta cell has reduced proliferative capacity, and in people with diabetes this is further confounded by higher rates of cellular apoptosis. Mechanisms underlying age-dependent reductions in the proliferation of beta cells include the reduced expression of activators of the cell cycle, increased expression of inhibitors of the cell cycle, and increased aggregation of amylin. Studying the aging pancreas in nondiabetic rodents and humans is a developing field, and therefore few broad conclusions can be drawn at this time.

The Aging Liver and Gallbladder

Next to skin and skeletal muscle, the liver is the largest organ in humans. In the average adult, the liver weighs about 1.2–1.5 kilograms (2.6–3.3 pounds) and constitutes about 2–5 percent of total body weight. The liver is strategically positioned in the systemic circulatory system to receive two sources of blood supply. Its supply of arterial blood comes through the hepatic artery, which represents about 25 percent of total hepatic blood flow. However, its largest volume of blood flow, nearly 75 percent of the total, comes from the portal vein. The portal vein contains an admixture of venous blood from the stomach, the small and large intestines, the pancreas, and the spleen. Physiologically, the liver's roles are diverse: it serves as a chemical modifications and productions factory, an excretory system, and both an endocrine and an exocrine gland. Because of its venous portal blood supply, the liver plays a key role in processing energy substrates that come from the foods we eat.

The functional anatomy and morphology of the liver are complex and beyond the scope of this book. In brief, liver lobules consist of hepatocytes, or liver cells; liver sinusoids, or unusually large capillaries with porous walls; and the intrahepatic biliary system, including the gallbladder (which is the source of concentration and storage of bile). Liver lobules are arranged hexagonally, and each lobule contains a central portal vein. At the apices of any two sides of each hexagon, there is a portal triad that consists of a branch of the hepatic artery, a branch of the portal vein, and a bile duct. These structures lie in close proximity to each other, which facilitates their physiological functions. Hepatocytes serve to detoxify, filter, inactivate, and metabolize a wide range of endogenous and exogenous substances that include aging red blood cells, bacteria, drugs, endotoxins, hormones, parasites, particulate matter, and other pathogens.

In addition, the liver is host to an abundance of fixed macrophages and phagocytes (Kupffer's cells) and therefore plays an important role in the immune system. Kupffer's cells make up 80–90 percent of the fixed macrophages. The liver also has the capacity to convert important hormones, minerals, and vitamins into more active forms—for example, by removing iodine from thyroxine (T4) to convert it to triiodothyronine (T3) and by adding the initial hydroxyl group to vitamin D. Furthermore, hepatic enzymes convert lipid-like compounds to more water-soluble forms that can be readily excreted in the bile. The liver stores carbohydrates (such as glycogen), lipids, minerals, and vitamins and synthesizes carbohydrates (hepatic gluconeogenesis), proteins (from recirculated amino acids), and products of intermediary metabolism.

Metabolically, the liver is a synthetic factory of important organic molecules. It extracts amino acids from dietary proteins and uses them to produce functional proteins that serve as transporters; colloids; and hemostatic, angiogenic, and growth factors. Circulating transport or binding proteins include those that carry copper, iron, vitamins, steroids, and other physiologically important molecules. Colloids include albumin and globulins that play essential roles in maintaining circulating blood volume and capillary hemodynamics. Hemostatic proteins are necessary for blood coagulation and antithrombosis. Angiogenic proteins and growth factors such as vascular endothelial growth factor help synthesize new blood vessels. The liver is critical to the physiology of lipid metabolism because it plays major roles in extracting, storing, and synthesizing triglycerides, cholesterol, free fatty acids, chylomicrons, and other products of the digestion or absorption of dietary lipids. The liver helps regulate circulating concentrations of triglycerides and is the primary site for the metabolism and storage of fat-soluble vitamins such as A, D, E, and K.

Bile is a complex physiological suspension; it is produced by the liver and stored in the gallbladder. Bile or biliary secretions have two main functions. They help remove important waste products such as bilirubin and cholesterol from the body, and they are essential to the digestion and absorption of dietary lipids. Epithelial cells that line the bile ducts perform important modifications of the bile as a result of their absorptive and secretory properties. Moreover, bile salts and bile pigments are concentrated inside the gallbladder as a result of their special circulation and recirculation and storage (reticuloendothelial circulation).

The reticuloendothelial circulation is a system for recycling bile that consists of its secretion by the liver and reabsorption by the intestinal tract, followed by the return of the unused bile to the liver via the hepatic portal blood for recirculation. The design of this physiological system of waste management and recycling is thousands of years old and far superior to synthetic systems. Our artificial systems of recycling didn't develop until after the founding of the Environmental Protection Agency in the early 1970s. In fact my area of central New Jersey, a national leader in recycling programs, did not pay serious attention to recycling until the mid-1990s or later. This is surprising, considering that New Jersey is the most densely populated state in the United States as well as the wealthiest (as measured by the number of millionaires living here as well as per capita) and is commonly characterized as the residence of forward-thinking people. Unfortunately, many municipalities in the United States still do not recycle.

The formation of bile occurs discretely and systematically. First, each liver cell actively secretes bile into apposed tiny channels called canaliculi. The newly formed bile is then transported by a system of intra- and extrahepatic bile ducts that secrete an aqueous, bicarbonate-rich fluid into the bile. These initial steps in the average adult can produce up to a liter of bile each day. In a third step between successive meals, approximately half of this hepatic bile is diverted into the gallbladder, where it is stored and concentrated by the removal of water and salts. Bile acids and bile salts can be concentrated ten- to twentyfold by the gallbladder before bile is released into the duodenum. These include bile salts, bilirubin, cholesterol, and lecithin. This means that the bile entering the small intestine is a mixture of relatively dilute hepatic bile and rather concentrated gallbladder bile. Improper diet and hydration over prolonged periods of time can disturb the balance of the formation and use of bile. Such disturbances often appear in the form of gallstones.

The flow of bile and the synthesis of bile salts are reduced by about 50 percent during the aging process, and the prevalence of gallstones rises with age. In addition, the sensitivity of the gallbladder to contractions stimulated by the hormone cholecystokinin also appears to decrease with age, while the volume of bile expelled in a twenty-four-hour period and the rate of emptying of the gallbladder are not affected. Perhaps the most compelling evidence for the maintenance of sufficient hepatic and gallbladder function into advanced age comes from clinical practice, in which donor livers from eighty-year-olds have been harvested and successfully transplanted into much younger recipients.

With old age, the liver also undergoes brown atrophy. Brown atrophy means the liver accumulates nonmetabolized proteins or pigmented waste products. The major such product is the wear-and-tear substance lipofuscin, which is an end product of fat metabolism in subcellular organelles. Another age-related change is a substantial reduction in total blood flow of about 40 percent. This has been documented in both humans and rodents. Because hepatic arterial blood supply as a proportion of cardiac output does not change with age (except in extreme conditions such as shock and trauma), and because there are no major changes in portal venous hemodynamics with age, the reduction in total hepatic blood flow is probably caused by diminished splanchnic blood flow, which would reduce venous drainage into the portal vein. This means that with age, the blood supply to the spleen, the pancreas, the small or large intestines, or all of these splanchnic organs could decrease.

Bile flow and the formation of bile salts are also reduced with age by an estimated 50 percent, and the hepatic synthesis of proteins, lipids, and glucose decreases with age as well. Total protein synthesis is reduced by about 50 percent in aging rats, a change that might be associated with impaired hepatic degradation of proteins or lack of availability of amino acids. In one study of about 11,000 humans, investigators found that plasma albumin decreased by about 10 percent with age (about 0.5 grams per liter per decade). In addition to the reductions in blood supply and the flow of bile, antioxidant activity in the liver appears to decline with age. This can be explained by the age-related reductions in the synthesis of hepatic antioxidant enzymes such as superoxide dismutase and glutathione peroxidase.

The effects of age on the liver's metabolic functions are of the utmost importance because elderly people are the most medicated subpopulation of our society, and because many if not most drugs are processed and eliminated by the liver. Unlike renal clearance, there is no well-developed scheme for quantitatively determining the clearance of drugs by the liver. The contribution of age to altered hepatic clearance of drugs is difficult to assess because drug interactions, numbers and types of drugs taken at a time, underlying disease, and increased individual variability are superimposed on the aging process. Therefore, changes in liver function with age mean potential impairment of the metabolism of drugs and their dangerous accumulation in the circulation and tissues of the elderly. Because of this, physicians prescribing drugs for the elderly need to take into consideration the decline in liver function. After much research into the matter, it seems that the well-known aphorism "start lower and go slower" is more valid than ever in the field of prescribing medications for the geriatric population. A general rule of thumb is: in the elderly, all drugs should be prescribed at starting doses that are 30–40 percent lower than the average dose used in middle-aged and younger adults.

Resting and Basal Metabolic Rates and Conclusion

Metabolism encompasses all the chemical processes involved in the growth of the body and in its production and use of energy. In a seventy-kilogram man, 2,100 calories per day are needed to support these activities. This is referred to as the resting metabolic rate. The basal metabolic rate, a clinical term, is different from the resting metabolic rate and is more rigidly defined. The basal metabolic rate is the number of calories consumed by a person who meets the following conditions: (1) having had a full night of restful sleep; (2) being in a neutral thermal environment (the temperature is not above or below the norm); (3) having fasted for at least twelve hours; (4) having been lying down and resting quietly for at least sixty minutes when the measurements are made; and (5) being free from psychological and physical stimuli. The units for basal metabolic rate are expressed in calories or kilocalories per hour or per square meters of body surface area. The basal metabolic rate is less than the resting metabolic rate and is about 5 percent less in women than in men.

In classic experiments designed to test the effects on eating behavior and metabolism of either electrically stimulating or damaging selective regions of the brain, researchers identified two areas of the hypothalamus that are important in controlling eating: a satiety center (dealing with eating satisfaction and cessation) and a hunger center (controlling feeding or eating behavior). Electrical stimulation of the satiety center makes an animal feel satisfied even when underfed and/or in the presence of food. Damaging this center leads to the continuous consumption of food even in the absence of need. Electrical stimulation of the hunger center leads to a voracious appetite even after the animal has ingested adequate amounts of food. Destroying the hunger center leads to complete and lasting cessation of the intake of food. The two centers combined control food consumption and therefore influence metabolism and body weight.

We are just beginning to understand the roles of the gastrointestinal and central nervous systems in controlling body weight with age. Our knowledge is expanding in large part due to modern parabiotic experiments in mice—experiments in which the circulatory systems of two mice are surgically connected, so they share about 1 percent of each other's blood supply. Actually, such donor or recipient experiments were developed by classic physiologists and pharmacologists many decades ago, first in donor organs and later in dogs. Only since the 1980s have such experiments been performed in mice, with the onset of the new era of modern molecular biology and the unraveling of the human and animal genomes.

One strain of mice used in parabiotic experiments is prone to obesity and is labeled the Ob/Ob strain. When given unlimited food, these mice become morbidly obese. They are typically at least 100 percent heavier than their unaffected littermates. When an Ob/Ob mouse and a normal littermate are exposed to the parabiotic experiment, the Ob/Ob mouse loses weight. This observation suggests that the Ob/Ob mouse is lacking a blood-borne factor that helps control body mass.

Another strain of mice that overeats develops diabetes in addition to obesity. Affected mice in this strain are labeled Db/Db. They also have adult body weights that are typically 100 percent greater than their unaffected littermates. When a Db/Db mouse and an unaffected littermate are studied parabiotically, the lean mouse starves. In a third kind of parabiotic experiment, an Ob/Ob and a Db/Db mice share the same circulation. Under these conditions, the Ob/Ob mouse loses weight, and the Db/Db mouse does not. Collectively, these results in obese mice suggest that: (1) the Db/Db mouse makes an excess of blood-borne factor that helps cure the Ob/Ob mouse; (2) the Db/Db mouse lacks the organ or tissue receptor for this factor; and (3) the absence of the receptor in the Db/Db mouse removes negative feedback, thus leading to high circulating concentrations of the blood-borne factor.

About two decades ago, investigators identified the blood-borne factor missing in Ob/Ob mice as leptin (from the Greek word for thin, *liptos*). The administration of leptin to Ob/Ob mice leads to rapid loss of weight. Unfortunately, results in humans have not been as promising. In the interim an appetite-enhancing factor, ghrelin, has been discovered, as mentioned above. In response to fasting, it is released by specialized cells in the stomach mucosa. Elevated plasma levels of ghrelin during fasting promote appetite and eating. Circulating concentrations of ghrelin are lower in obese than in lean humans, suggesting that it does not drive food intake in the obese. However, gastric bypasses in the moribundly obese cause marked reductions in circulating ghrelin as well as loss of weight and appetite.

Clearly, more work is needed to help us fully understand the roles of leptin, ghrelin, insulin, glucagon, and other blood-borne factors that influence the gastrointestinal system, appetite, and body mass during aging. In the meantime, self-control and moderation seem to be keys to maintaining a healthy body weight at any age. This behavior can and should be taught by parents to children, and by caregivers to those in their charge.

8

The Aging Musculoskeletal System

Between Thanksgiving to mid-December 2013, I discontinued my exercise routine. This was due to travel out-of-state, illness after I returned, and seasonal weather. During that period of little purposeful exercise, I cut down a neighbor's tree. The roots were threatening his swimming pool, and the tree's location was causing some contention with a third neighbor. The task took several hours, and I hadn't done this kind of activity for years. Several days later, the muscles in the region of the little and ring fingers of my left hand were sore and almost unusable. I had strained muscle and other soft tissues that were not used to that kind of work. This further delayed my return to my routine schedule of physical activity, which includes bench presses, since I couldn't grip the bar or lift the weight.

Perhaps the strain would not have been so evident had I been younger. However, I prefer to think it was due almost exclusively to my failure to use a chain saw routinely. In any event, I paid a price for engaging in the activity but felt compensated for having helped a couple of neighbors in need.

Types and Organization of Muscle

A complete classification of the muscles in humans is beyond the scope of this book. However, it is instructive for readers to have some knowledge of muscle tissue, how it is organized, and how it functions. This will help as you read this chapter and learn more about the effects of aging on muscle and bony structures of the body.

Consider your biceps. Beneath the skin and subcutaneous tissue each bicep is contained in an external, delimiting sheath called the epimysium. The bicep can be further subdivided into muscle fascicles that are contained in sheaths called perimysiums (perimysia). Fascicles, bundles of similarly sized muscles, consist of muscle fibers that are each delineated by an endomysium sheath. Each of the muscle fibers (muscle cells, or myocytes) is surrounded by a plasma membrane called the sarcolemma. In addition, each muscle fiber contains many myofibrils, which are end-to-end chains of repeating units called sarcomeres. Sarcomeres consist of smaller, interdigitating filaments called myofilaments. In turn, each myofilament is composed of thick and thin filaments.

The sarcomere is both the structural and functional unit of striated skeletal and cardiac muscle (in humans and other mammals, the vast majority of striated muscle is skeletal). The smallest contractile unit of striated muscle is the multinucleated, elongated muscle cell. Striated muscle, both skeletal and cardiac, was given its name because the repeating units of sarcomeres and the thick and thin filaments that compose them give the appearance of striations when the muscle is viewed under a light or electron microscope.

Striated skeletal muscle can also be divided into slow- and fast-twitch classes. Slow-twitch or type I myocytes develop force slowly when stimulated and also relax slowly. Fast-twitch muscle fibers develop force in shorter periods of time and also relax more rapidly. Slow-twitch myocytes are further referred to as oxidative, while fast-twitch myocytes are called glycolytic. Slow-twitch muscles do not fatigue easily because they have many capillaries, mitochondria, and myoglobin (red color–enhancing muscle protein); fast-twitch muscles lack these properties and do fatigue easily. However, fast-twitch myocytes rely on their own storage of glycogen for energy and can move heavier loads in shorter periods of time than slow-twitch myocytes. In contrast, slow-twitch muscle cells use glucose and free fatty acids provided by the circulation and move lighter loads over longer periods of time.

In addition to striated muscle, our bodies contain another kind of muscle called nonstriated. This is smooth muscle, which can be subclassified as either vascular or visceral smooth muscle. Vascular smooth muscle cells line the walls of arteries and veins. Visceral smooth muscle is found in the walls of other tubular organs such as the gastrointestinal tract, oviducts in women, and the vas deferens in men. Smooth muscle cells are not as highly organized as striated muscle cells, but both kinds of cells can shorten and generate force in response to physiological stimuli. Both kinds are also innervated and subject to the influences of the central, peripheral, and autonomic nervous systems. Therefore, decline in muscle function with age is codependent on declines in function of the central nervous system, particularly the motor cortex.

Motor Cortex and Muscle Function with Age

Aging is associated with marked reductions in muscle strength and motor control. Many of the changes in muscle function result from adaptations to aging that take place in the central nervous system. For example, aging is associated with broad qualitative and quantitative changes in the motor cortex. Among these are cortical atrophy, reduced cortical excitability, impaired cortical plasticity, and imbalances in neurotransmitters. Tissue sections of humans who died without signs of neurological disease suggest that people over sixty-five years of age, in comparison to adults younger than forty-five, have a 43 percent reduction in the volume of cell bodies of neurons in the premotor cortex. These early observations in cadavers have been corroborated more recently in live humans using high-resolution magnetic resonance imaging (MRI).

MRIs obtained from 106 cognitively sound individuals ranging in age from eighteen to ninety-three years revealed that thinning of the cortex occurs by middle age, and that areas near the primary motor cortex (for example, the precentral gyrus) demonstrate prominent atrophy with age. Moreover, changes in the size of the motor cortex and age-related differences in the mass of white matter and in the length of myelinated neurons also exist. Specifically, among people eighteen to ninety-three years of age whose deaths were unrelated to deficits in the nervous system, the length of myelinated nerve fibers in cortical white matter decreased by 45 percent with age.

In addition to age-related morphological changes in the brain, neurochemical changes in the basal ganglia that control coordination, movement, and other motor functions have been of great interest to investigators. Once scientists learned that depletion of the neurotransmitter dopamine underlies the motor deficits in Parkinson's disease, the field of neurotransmitters and age mushroomed. For several decades, age-related changes in neurotransmitters and their receptors have been associated with impaired cognition and motor functions. Indeed, impaired neurotransmission is responsible for at least some of the behavioral abnormalities associated with aging. This is illustrated by age-related changes in at least six or seven neurotransmitter-receptor systems, as well as corresponding reductions in neurotrophic factors in the motor cortex.

Such age-related changes in the dopaminergic system are perhaps the best understood of those in neurotransmitter systems because of dopamine's involvement in manual dexterity. Older adults exhibit reduced availability of dopamine transporters, and aging rodents have decreased dopamine-D2 receptors. The messenger RNA for this particular receptor is reduced by 50 percent in older animals. More recently, scientists have begun to examine interactions among multiple neurotransmitters and their receptors. Age-related changes in the interactions between dopamine, glutamate, and gamma amino butyric acid in regions of the central nervous system that govern emotions, motor behavior, and motivation might be associated with the choice of the elderly to engage in less physical activity.

The effect of aging on excitability in the cortex has been examined using transcranial magnetic stimulation. This is an experimental technique that allows the investigator to assess facilitation and inhibition in the motor cortex. Results of one recent investigation suggest that middle-aged adults have reduced cortical excitability in comparison to younger adults. That is, people in their late fifties through early sixties show more intracortical inhibition and less intracortical facilitation than do young adults in their twenties. Other findings in people with a mean age of seventy-one years support these results.

Motor tasks that activate sensorimotor regions of the brain are also affected by age. For example, functional MRIs have been used to quantify changes in cerebral blood flow and oxygenation as an indirect measure of neural activity during the performance of given motor tasks. Results reveal that older adults exhibit additional activation in areas that perform sensory and motor processing during these tasks, particularly on the side of the brain that is stimulated by the test. One such investigation focused on the effects of aging on oxygenation and cerebral blood flow during hand-grip contractions of varying intensities. The investigators observed that the motor cortex of older adults was less able to increase its activity when greater handgrip force was required.

In addition to age-related decrements in excitability and activity, the human motor cortex is also characterized by an age-dependent reduction in cortical functions such as creating new neurons. One group of investigators reported that the incremental electrical stimulation of a wrist nerve caused an increased amplitude of corresponding action potentials in motor nerves in young and middle-aged adults (ages twenty-one to fifty-nine years) but not in those ages sixty years and older. These investigators did not report data for the strength of corresponding muscle contractions (for example, finger twitches that could have been evoked by stimulating a nerve in the wrist). Still, the above findings confirm that aging results in reduced excitability in the motor cortex, a loss of functional asymmetry, reduced ability to modulate the activity of inappropriate motor networks when required, and attenuated cortical function, all of which probably contribute to age-related reductions in motor performance.

Aging and Maximal Voluntary Muscle Contraction

Aging is commonly associated with muscle weakness. The loss of muscle strength is likely due to a wide variety of physiological mechanisms, including reductions in muscle mass and changes in the excitation-contraction coupling process. Excitation-contraction coupling is the interaction between an excited motor nerve and the muscle fibers it attaches to. Normally, when the nerve fires, the muscle contracts. It is also probable that some fraction of the loss in muscle strength is due to cortical mechanisms and the nervous system's inability to fully activate skeletal muscle.

With aging, the loss of muscle strength is substantially greater than the loss of muscle mass. This dissociation suggests that explanatory mechanisms other than muscle atrophy influence the decrement in strength. Reductions in muscle strength but not muscle mass are independently associated with the development of disabilities, reduced functional capacity, and even increased risk of mortality. The associated physiological effects influence numerous aspects of muscle performance such as endurance and motor control. More specifically, there is reduced excitability in the motor cortex and spinal cord. Other changes include altered discharge properties of motor units, reduced numbers and sizes of motor units, changes in membrane excitability and thresholds for stimulation, slowing in the formation and cycling of cross-bridges (molecular connections between thick and thin filaments in sarcomeres), and decreased stiffness in tendons. It is irrefutable that aging causes marked reductions in these qualities of muscle function. This makes it imperative that investigators understand the role of the central nervous system in mediating the age-dependent loss of muscle strength.

Researchers have recently observed that in people with mild cognitive impediments, poor physical function and weakened muscle strength coexist. They have also noted that this relationship is independent of muscle mass and a person's level of physical activity. Theoretically, such changes in the motor cortex would reduce maximal force of voluntary muscle contraction. This would occur because of the physiological properties explained above, such as reduced excitation-contraction coupling or reduced number and size of motor units. Also, muscle weakness associated with aging is partially due to impairments in the nervous system's ability to fully activate motor neurons, particularly in the larger proximal muscle groups such as the elbow flexors and the knee extensors. The examples are clinically important because these muscles move heavy loads (for example, arms and elbows lifting Thanksgiving turkeys, and knees and legs moving furniture).

Data from a recent longitudinal study of aging reveal that muscle strength decreases at the staggering rate of 3 percent per year between the ages of seventy and seventy-nine. The resultant muscle weakness is independently associated with the development of disability, impairment of functional capacity, risk of falling and breaking bones, and even mortality. Consider, for example, former president George H. W. Bush, who not long ago was skydiving, but who in 2013 started using a motorized wheelchair to get around.

In June 2013 my wife and I attended our first senior prom in many years. This was no ordinary senior prom. Attendees were some of the senior citizens of our township who had been born in the months of April, May, and June and were being honored by the mayor and town council.

I estimated that about one hundred seniors were in attendance, eighty or ninety of whom were women. The oldest attendee had just turned ninety-six. Others were in their late seventies to mid-eighties. Some came with walkers or in wheelchairs. The event began with dinner (which started at 4:30 P.M.) and brief remarks by the mayor. There was a DJ who must have been about seventy-five but who could still sing, play the keyboard, and use karaoke as backup. Dancing began about 5:30–6:00 P.M., and the undesignated king and queen of the prom moved slowly onto the dance floor. No more than ten or fifteen different dancers, mostly women, were on the floor for any given song. The men who were able to move only waltzed. I imagined that most attendees thought of years gone by and of their days as teenagers when they could cut the rug with the best of other dancers. The prom ended at 7:30 P.M. so the honorees could return home and get to bed by 8:00.

That senior prom was a memorable event for several reasons. It was the first such activity for my wife and me. Father's Day and our anniversary were the following Sunday and Monday. It was a privilege being in the company of hepta-, octa-, and nonagenarians even if for only a few hours. At the university I have been surrounded by twenty-year-olds for nearly forty years. The change was a breath of fresh air. As long as we live nearby, we will probably become permanent attendees at the annual North Brunswick seniors' senior prom.

Physical Competition and Musculoskeletal Health

Osteoporosis is characterized by reduced density of minerals in bone and disrupted structure of bone. An estimated 10 million people in the United States have osteoporosis; most of them are elderly. Another 34 million are estimated to have osteopenia, which puts them at an increased risk of osteoporosis. The characteristic of reduced bone density increases the risk of fracturing bones. Fifty percent of women and about half this percentage of men over age fifty will suffer an osteoporosis-related fracture in their lifetime. Fracture of the hip will account for approximately 15 percent of these cases. Fractures of the hip are a leading cause of morbidity and mortality among the elderly. A recent Canadian investigation found that of 3,981 patients aged sixty years or older admitted to a hospital for fracture of the hip, 6 percent died in the hospital, and 31 percent—about one third of the cases studied—died within a year of the fracture. Few other demographics were given, but I assume most of these people were not Senior Olympians.

In July 2013, 10,888 registered athletes competed at the National Senior Games (the Senior Olympics) held in Cleveland, Ohio, and more than 25,000 spectators attended events. This was the greatest participation by athletes and spectators in the games' fourteen-year history. The Senior Olympics is an eighteen sport competition that is held in odd-numbered years. Athletes qualify for the Senior Olympics by winning events in their individual states' senior games. The eighteen sports are archery, badminton, basketball, bowling, cycling, golf, horseshoes, race walking, racquetball, road racing, shuffleboard, softball, swimming, table tennis, tennis, track and field, a triathlon, and volleyball. Of these, basketball, road racing, track and field, the triathlon, and volleyball are considered high-impact sports due to the almost continuous running and jumping involved. The remaining thirteen events are classified as non-high-impact or low-impact sports.

Gymnastics, weight lifting, and wrestling were not part of the most recent Senior Olympics. One of my sons was a good wrestler in high school, and I follow the Rutgers University wrestling team each year. I can't imagine the brittle bones and scrawny arms and legs of Senior Olympians withstanding the strains and stresses of the pretzel-like knots wrestlers often find themselves tied in. In fact, wrestling is one sport I would not approve for anyone older than about thirty years. There are others as well.

Having said that, I will note that gymnastics, weight lifting, and wrestling are all known to improve agility and balance, muscle mass and strength, and bone density. To perform well in international competition, wrestlers of any age have to achieve an excellent level of physical fitness during training. In general, successful wrestlers show higher dynamic (walking, running) and passive strength (weight-bearing activities) than unsuccessful wrestlers. Specifically, upper body strength and aerobic power are significantly different between the two groups. Aerobic capacity, or the ability to ventilate one's lungs, is one of the most important physiological factors for achieving successful results in competitive wrestling—or indeed any physical activity.

The maximum uptake of oxygen in wrestlers who compete internationally is near 50–60 milliliters per kilogram per minute (values of 70 or more are reported in endurance runners). Flexibility among wrestlers is lower than that among weight lifters and gymnasts, even though all three activities are known to increase muscle strength, flexibility, and endurance. Hypothetically, these activities are as applicable to the elderly as they are to the young. Still, prudence and wisdom should guide one's decision about whether or not to perform any physical activity.

From about the age of forty, men and women lose on average half of a percent of their bone mass each year. Evidence suggests that high-impact exercise can reduce the risk of falling in older people if the physical activities include exercises to improve balance, leg strength, and flexibility or endurance training. Consistent with these notions, one study found that among Senior Olympians, participation in high-impact sports was associated with a higher density of minerals in bones, whereas a lower density was associated with increased age, being a woman, and having been diagnosed by a physician as obese. Therefore, high-impact exercise (for example, a Zumba workout at reduced intensity) might prove to be a valuable activity for reducing the morbidity and mortality associated with fractures of the hip in the elderly.

Mobility and Muscle Power in the Aging

Preventing, postponing, and minimizing the limitations in mobility for the aging population is a major public health concern. Mobility, defined simply as the ability to move and get around with limited assistance, is essential to independent living. Limitations in mobility—reasonably defined as difficulty in performing what should be routine physical tasks such as walking short distances (several hundred yards to a quarter of a mile) without help or without being exhausted, climbing three or four flights of stairs (ascending 25–30 feet), or getting up from a chair or sofa— are indicative of a marked decline in functional health. The best evidence that the above definitions are valid is the thousands of older people who can do these things and more because they are determined.

For a time during his twenty-first year, my son was stationed with the Marine Corps in Brooklyn. He held the annual physical fitness record among recruits for doing the most pull-ups. However, one of his noncommissioned officers, a seventy-year-old master sergeant or sergeant major, could outperform him in this event. This older man was a fit role model for my son and others like him. He worked out regularly, watched his diet, and aimed to make physical fitness a permanent part of his life. Oorah!

A growing body of literature has established reductions in muscle strength—that is, the ability to generate maximal muscle force—as a leading cause of functional deficit in the elderly. However, skeletal muscle power—or the product of the force and velocity of muscle contraction—has been shown to decline earlier and more rapidly than muscle strength with advancing age. The underlying physiological mechanisms that contribute to the reduction in muscle power in older adults include: (1) sarcopenia; (2) changes in muscle composition or types of fibers; (3) reduced muscle strength per unit of muscle mass; (4) changing contractile properties of individual muscle fibers; and (5) alterations at the neuromuscular junction that affect synaptic transmission and the binding of neurotransmitters to motor endplates.

In recent years, some investigators have been focusing on muscle power in the lower extremities as a more critical variable in understanding the relationship between impairments, functional limitations, and resultant immobility in the elderly. These investigators feel that peak muscle power (as opposed to muscle strength) is a more reliable predictor of functional performance in older adults. Muscle power can be assessed using a wide range of external resistances. External resistance is the force a muscle must work against in order to lift a load. Such resistance can be adjusted to some percentage (for example, 50–100 percent) of that calculated when a load or weight is lifted a single time. This has been called the one repetition maximum resistance. Under these conditions, peak muscle power is typically identified at approximately 70 percent of the value for one repetition maximum resistance. Conversely, the maximum velocity of contraction routinely occurs at the lowest external resistance, or at 40 percent. Muscle strength, on the other hand, represents the greatest load (weight) lifted during a test of the one repetition maximum.

Muscle function can also be reliably assessed using dynamometry. A dynamometer is a mechanical or electrical instrument that is used to test the strength of one's grip. One's grip is a measure of the strength of hand

and forearm muscles. These same devices are used to evaluate muscle fatigue. Fatigue, in this case, is the decline in strength or force observed over time as one tries to maintain an initial grip. My colleagues and I in the Systems Physiology Laboratory at Rutgers University use dynamometers to help teach advanced undergraduates the physiology of human skeletal muscle.

Additional methods that have been used to evaluate power in the lower extremities of older people include jumping vertically on a force platform and rapidly extending the lower limbs without moving a load. The more recent use of pneumatic resistance training equipment in the elderly has emerged as an accurate and valid assessment tool. Unlike some techniques, this methodology consistently and more reliably captures both the components of force and velocity of muscle power. Experimental protocols allowing the elderly to make multiple attempts at achieving maximum velocity of contraction and therefore maximal muscle power are useful even in the frailest among us.

Factors that lead to a reduction in the force and/or velocity of contraction contribute to reduced muscle power with advancing age. These factors include sarcopenia and a selective reduction in the number and size of type II muscle fibers, which have four times the power-generating ability of type I fibers. Additionally, loss of muscle power in older adults is influenced by the infiltration of muscle by fat, the changing architecture of muscle, the reduced synthesis of muscle proteins, mediators of inflammation, and changing hormonal status (for example, lower testosterone). Still, a distinct physiological basis for the precipitous decline in muscle power with aging has yet to be identified, and additional research should focus on clarifying the relationship between impairments in muscle power and the onset of limitations in mobility associated with aging. In any case, activities designed to improve power in the arms and hands, legs and feet, shoulders, back, and abdomen are effective in younger people and should be safe and well tolerated in older adults.

The Aging Shoulders

Dysfunction and disease of the shoulder are growing concerns not only for the aging population, but also for athletes and laborers. Osteoarthritis of the shoulder and diseases of or injury to the rotator cuff represent the two most common disorders of the shoulder that lead to degeneration, disability, discomfort, and pain. Stem cell research as it might apply to the regeneration of the cartilage of joints has not yet been translated from the basic science laboratory to the clinic. Still, the fields of shoulder orthroscopic surgery and orthroplasty have advanced to the point that joint replacement is an excellent and viable option for a number of pathologic conditions in the shoulder. Also, treating maladies of the rotator cuff has been a significant focus of research in recent years because of poor healing of tendons and irreversible changes associated with injury to the rotator cuff.

As the size of the elderly population increases, so do the rates of age-related orthopedic disorders. This is of particular concern in the field of shoulder pathology because both osteoarthritis and diseases of the rotator cuff are degenerative conditions that increase with age. These conditions represent the most common causes of pain and disability in the shoulder and have been the subjects of innovation in research and treatment in recent years. Any number of events can cause arthritis of the shoulder. Lack of blood flow and death of tissue, infection, inflammation, osteoarthritis, and trauma can all lead to the loss of integrity of cartilage and to the destruction of the surfaces of joints. Loss of or damage to cartilage (tears) and the development of incompatible surfaces of the joint can result in painful articulation that requires orthopedic surgery.

Osteoarthritis is the most common cause of shoulder discomfort and disease and has been linked to both age and chronic overuse. Options for conventional treatment include nonsteroidal anti-inflammatory drugs (taken orally), steroid injections such as triamcinolone acetate, orthroscopic debridement, and replacement of the joint. It is expected that the rate of orthroplasty of the arm and shoulder will soon double, helping increase the costs of health care and imposing additional economic burdens on society as a whole. Diseases and disabilities of the rotator cuff are age-dependent and exist along a spectrum from tendinitis through partial-thickness tears to full-thickness tears.

A recent study demonstrated that 21 percent of the people in a Japanese village had tears of the rotator cuff. In this study, risk factors for tearing the rotator cuff included a history of trauma of the shoulder or upper arm, use of the dominant arm, and age. Other investigators have reported that in shoulders free of disease and pain, an increased prevalence of tears is associated with increased age. Moreover, tears can enlarge over time, and the increasing size of the tear is accompanied by the retraction of the associated muscle-tendon unit. This leads to changes in the morphology of the muscle, misalignment of the joint, and altered biomechanics. Not all tears of the rotator cuff are painful, but repair of painful tears is one of the most common orthopedic procedures in the United States.

In general, degenerative conditions of the shoulder and upper arm remain a significant source of pain and disability in the general and elderly populations. The burden of arthritis and diseases of the rotator cuff make the conditions prime topics for basic translational research. Although total shoulder replacement remains the last resort for treating severe disorders of the shoulder, other therapies are on the horizon. Research on the tendon has focused on preventing failures of repairs to the rotator cuff and augmenting the physiological healing of the tissue. Many potential therapies hold promise, and the implementation of new technologies such as bioengineered scaffolding, novel sources of stem cells, and controlled-release of tissue growth factors will likely become more broadly available in the future.

Because of continuous physical activity, I've had orthoscopic surgery—not on my shoulders, but on both knees. These were uncomplicated, outpatient procedures to remove bone fragments and trim torn cartilage. On one such occasion I complained to my orthopedist about recent and sustained pain in my posterior right shoulder. After answering his questions, I asked what could be done. He recommended some stretching exercises and said if the pain didn't stop he would give me a steroid injection. Four to six weeks of the prescribed exercises did not alleviate the pain, so he gave me the injection. He administered about forty milligrams in 1–2 milliliters of a liquid solution of triamcinolone acetate (Kenalog, 40 mg i.m.). Within a few days the pain was gone, and I had greater mobility and range of motion in my right shoulder for the next couple of years.

That first experience occurred in 2003. My latest injection of triamcinolone acetate (50 mg i.m.) was administered in December 2010, by my family physician (who is experienced in sports medicine and the treatment of injured athletes). This injection was given in the left anterior shoulder. The pain was relieved a few days later, and I have not needed steroid injections since. Both physicians concluded that the cause of my pain was inflammation at the sites of muscle insertion into bone.

Between 2003 and 2010, I had four or five such injections. These experiences and my desire to minimize the need for future injections taught me a lesson. I began using my shoulders more frequently. After arising and showering (I get up between 4:00 and 6:00 A.M.), I do fifty military-style push-ups. I then roll onto my back and do 100 abdominal crunches. The push-ups take about one minute and the crunches three or four more because I add leg lifts. The crunches are unorthodox because I use them as much for my shoulders as for my abdominal muscles. When I do each crunch, I pretend to pump air into a bicycle tire. This forces me to keep my shoulders and arms moving during those few minutes.

After the push-ups and crunches, I do two or three sets of bench presses, using about 100 pounds. Each set consists of eight to twelve repetitions. Including periods of rest, this weight-lifting activity takes another eight to ten minutes. Following the bench presses, I do a similar series of butterflies, using about 35 pounds in each hand (another eight to ten minutes). This early morning shoulder-and-arm routine has made it possible for me to avoid any further discomfort, pain, or steroid injections in both shoulders. Additional benefits are increased strength and power in my shoulders and upper arms.

To supplement my shoulder and upper-arm exercises, during the period April through November I push my lawnmower and use my edger and weed whacker to maintain our lawns and property. I have provided my own yard service for nearly fifty years. I also wash, dry, and detail our cars on a regular basis. These activities ensure that I make adequate use of my arms, shoulders, and back. There is inadequate space here to enumerate all the other benefits I am aware of.

The Aging Feet and Footwear

Both arthritis and pain in the feet are major public health problems. An estimated 24 percent of adults have ailments of the feet, and the prevalence increases with age. The shoes we wear and footwear-related pain are most definitely modifiable behaviors. However, arthritis and rheumatic disorders of the foot might not be, and it is surprising that this topic has received little attention in the rheumatology community.

My mother, a younger sister, and I have all suffered from ingrown toenails. The women's cases were much more serious than mine and led to the complete removal of nails. My sister eventually had distal bone removed from both large toes, and soft tissue sutured from top and bottom to form thumb-like stubs. I suspect that most of this was due to our footwear, our ages, and paying too much attention to fashion. The damage was done in our teenage years.

In February 1964 the Beatles came to the United States for their first of several live performances. Ed Sullivan hosted them on his CBS television variety show in Manhattan. Among several other distinguishing characteristics of the Beatles were tight-legged slacks and pointed-toed shoes (later called Beatle boots). I was an impressionable teenager and had to have a pair of Beatle boots. I had not had ingrown toenails before I began wearing those shoes. Also, young men in the area where I lived at the time wore two pairs of socks, one over the other. These were no ordinary cotton or thin nylon socks. They were thick, woolly, and resembled ski socks. Needless to say, the shoes and socks crowded my feet and pinched my toes. Moreover, skinny jeans that teenagers and young adults are wearing as I write (in 2013 and 2014) were also fashionable in the mid-1960s after the onset of Beatlemania, and I began wearing them. During this time, our family relocated to a different state. My fashions were not in vogue in my new high school, and my dress standard must have created more than one or two snickers and sneers. It also resulted in unwelcome visits to the principal's office. Pegged-leg jeans that could barely fit over double-layered socks and Beatle boots made me stand out in every crowd—in school corridors and at football games and dances. It was in this new community and after about one year that my toenails became ingrown and infected. Fortunately, a kind but firm family physician told me my toe problems were caused by my shoes and socks. He advised me to change, and I did.

My next bout with foot-related pain came some thirty years later, when I developed heel spurs from too much running on hard paved surfaces. Soon thereafter I became aware of the potential role of footwear and orthotics in the treatment of rheumatoid and osteoarthritis of the hip, knee, and foot. Despite the great amount of attention that has been paid to the structure and alignment of bones and joints in arthritis, surprisingly little work has been devoted to the foot. Evidence from biomechanical experiments indicates that foot orthotics and specialized footwear can change the activation of muscles and the patterns of gaits. Such changes can also potentially reduce the loads placed on the bones, joints, and soft tissue of the feet.

As the number of older adults increases, so too will the economic and societal burdens caused by problems of the feet and lower limbs. For example, responses to a podiatric supplement to the US National Health Interview Survey led to estimates that 24 percent of the population have at least one foot ailment, and that older adults are more affected than younger ones. Moreover, recent data from the Framingham Heart Study found that 19 percent of men and 29 percent of women reported foot pain on most days of the month. The prevalence of pain at specific locations in the foot ranged from 7 percent to 13 percent. People suffering from rheumatoid arthritis have approximately twice the prevalence of foot pain as the general population does. Yet definitive data are sparse, and it is still premature for clinicians to recommend treatment.

During the past few decades, the procedure of bracing the osteoarthritic knee has attracted significant attention for its role in correcting misalignment of joints and reducing the osteoarthritis. In contrast, very little work has focused on interventions other than surgery that might benefit painful feet. The popular belief is that corrections for ailments of the foot using therapeutic footwear cause changes in alignment of the spine and pelvic girdle. Other research suggests that the benefit of foot orthotics and specialized shoes comes from changing the shank and activation of muscles of the foot (changing the gait). Correcting the distribution of weight on the feet and stabilizing the foot and ankle might reduce the likelihood of deformities and walking disabilities for patients with rheumatoid arthritis. This is commonly thought to be accomplished through the use of orthotics or custom footwear. However, reviews of these devices in patients with rheumatoid arthritis do not support their use, leading the authors of one review to report finding hardly any evidence in favor of prescribing custom-made foot orthotics for patients with rheumatoid arthritis.

The heel bone spurs that I mentioned above were caused by running, at least according to the orthopedists, podiatrists, and general practitioners I consulted at the time. Each of them recommended that I use orthotics to correct the problem. My health insurance did not cover that expense, so I began a search for shoe inserts that might help. On an experimental basis I went through several types, including gel-like heel caps. None of these helped. Then, in the mid-1990s, I found a type of heel cup that worked: my heel pain has not returned since I began wearing them. I use heel cups in dress shoes as well as sneakers, especially any time I will be on my feet for more than an hour. Two of our daughters have recently developed similar heel pain. One has been a nurse in neonatal intensive care units and has often been on her feet during twelve-hour shifts several times a week. I recommended heel cups to both daughters, and they too have had reduced pain since starting to use the cups.

Women tend to be at a greater risk of hip and knee osteoarthritis than men are, so shoes that women wear, particularly high heels, have been implicated in these conditions. Still, one retrospective analysis of osteoarthritis of the knee found that wearing high heels did not increase the risk for the disease. This report cast doubt on the belief that high heels are a major factor in promoting the degeneration of the knee joint in women. Many investigators have examined factors associated with painful feet in women, including the kinds of shoes they were wearing at the time and had worn in the past. Women who regularly wore high heels, sandals, and slippers in the past were more likely to experience pain in the feet in later years, compared to women who wore other types of footwear. Another study examined the prevalence of current pain among older Brazilian men and women when wearing shoes, and the relation between pain in the feet and wearing high heels. Women were more prone to pain in the feet than men (50 percent and 30 percent, respectively). In that study, currently wearing high heels was not associated with painful feet in women.

Though the long-term effects of wearing high heels are uncertain, wearing shoes in general correlates with poor alignment and development of the feet. Investigators who conducted a study of more than 4,000 Indians (adults and children) found that wearing shoes during the critical ages for the development of the foot's arch (up to six years) increased the incidence of flat feet. The longer a child waited before wearing shoes regularly, the less likely he or she was to have flat feet and problems with foot ligaments as an adult. Moreover, there is a known association between the structure of the foot and the development of osteoarthritis. Therefore, the history of one's footwear and the foot's current structure will likely become more important in understanding the progress of degenerative diseases of the knee joint and the role of the feet on these.

The Aging Hands and Fingers

On two separate occasions, my wife spent a few weeks with her aging father shortly before his death in 2010. During those visits, she observed his decreasing ability to take care of his personal hygiene. For example, he was unable to clip his toenails. This was probably compounded by aging-related discouragement and depression—increased by the recent death of his wife—and continuous pain in his lower legs. A general decline in manual dexterity is a phenomenon that is commonly observed in the elderly, who seem to have increasing difficulty in performing routine activities such as handling coins, preparing meals, and writing checks.

To confirm this perception, there are various standardized tasks used to test dexterity in the elderly. Individually and collectively, these tests demonstrate that older adults take more time than younger ones to complete such tasks. In addition to being slower, the elderly readjust their grasping of objects more often and demonstrate greater variations in patterns of grasping. For example, a younger adult might grasp an object using the thumb and forefinger, while an older person might grasp it using the thumb, forefinger, and middle finger (called a tripod pinch) or the thumb, ring finger, and little finger (known as a lateral pinch). In addition to the strength of muscles and the sensory and anatomical integrity of the hand and fingers, the effective handling of an object requires precision manipulation and temporal control of forces at the fingertips. One example is turning on an electric range and adjusting the temperature. The physiological sensorimotor responses involved in such actions have been investigated by examining forces at the fingertips during simple grasp, lift, and hold exercises. It should come as no surprise that a decline in manual dexterity impairs one's ability to live independently and thus increases the likelihood of being admitted to a nursing home.

The lifting and holding of an object is composed of four distinct phases: preload, loading, transitional, and static. During the preload phase, one's fingers contact the object and a small grip force, appropriate for the surface of the object, is applied before initiation of the force that will lift the load vertically. In the subsequent loading phase, the force of one's grip increases in proportion to the weight of the object. This force is applied until it exceeds the opposing forces of gravity, when the object is lifted. The transitional phase begins at lift-off and continues until the object is raised to its desired position. Grip and load forces reach their maximal values during this phase. The static phase is achieved one second after a stable grip is reached and the object is held at the new height. During lifting and holding, the magnitude of one's grip is adjusted to the object's weight, center of gravity, and frictional conditions at the interface between fingers and object (for example, tightening one's grip to hold onto a slippery object). If the force of one's grip is insufficient, one might lose hold of the object, causing it to fall. Conversely, excessive force of grip can result in premature fatigue of muscle, the crushing of fragile objects, or difficulties in manipulating the basic grasp.

Healthy young adults use forces of grip that are just slightly above those necessary to prevent the object from slipping. This is an energy-efficient method for maintaining the stability and security of the object. The healthy elderly use excessive gripping forces. Perhaps this is an acknowledgment of their weakened muscle condition or their fear of failing at the task. Moreover, forces of grip among the elderly are more variable than they are among younger adults. Increased force of grip is by far the most consistent age-related change in one's control of grasp. Forces of grip in the elderly are excessive during both static and dynamic tasks, and during continuous and discrete efforts. Comparing young subjects with older ones, researchers have consistently observed the increase in force among the elderly regardless of the properties of the object, the number of fingers involved, the ease or difficulty of the task, and whether participants were seated or standing. These effects of age begin as early as fifty years.

Increments in the force of one's grip during aging are thought to be a function of changes in the skin. Changes in the content and distribution of water could make the skin drier and, in turn, might affect friction at the interface between fingers and objects. This could lead to reduced ability in the elderly to handle objects and thus to dropping objects more frequently. This skin-hydration hypothesis is supported by studies showing that the minimum force required to prevent an object from slipping (the so-called slip force) increases as we age. However, I could find no studies comparing the force of grip between long-time residents of the Southwest versus Northeast. There is solid evidence that the skin of residents of southwestern states such as Arizona and New Mexico is less hydrated than that of counterparts in northeastern states such as New York and New Jersey.

Also with advancing age, the safety margin employed by the elderly is elevated, indicating an increase in the force of one's grip that exceeds the force necessary to compensate for increased slipperiness. This increased safety margin has been attributed to deterioration of sensory processing at the fingertips. Increasing the force of the grip and safety margin reduces the elderly person's dependence on sensory signals. Reductions in the number and size of mechanoreceptors at the fingertips also occur with aging. Moreover, sensory signals in the elderly are attenuated due to the increased threshold potentials that are needed to generate action potentials. Clinical evaluation of the function of mechanoreceptors in the hand reveals that the elderly typically have increased thresholds for detecting minimal mechanical forces at the fingertips and for detecting two-point discrimination. These limitations are correlated with deficits in manual dexterity, such as turning playing cards over and placing pegs in a pegboard. Such tests highlight the role of tactile sensation mediated by mechanoreceptors in tasks requiring manual dexterity.

The relationship between the force of one's grip and loss of sensory perception in the fingertips becomes progressively more evident in adults sixty years of age and older. When people in this age group participate in scientific studies, they use higher safety margins when the texture of an object's surface but not its weight is changed, indicating selectively impaired detection of friction. These participants also use a default force of grip based on the most slippery surface. Considered collectively, these findings imply that the age-related increase in the force of one's grip compensates for a reduction in tactile sensation in the fingertips and/or accompanying sensations of increasing slipperiness of objects. In either case, the strategy of gripping more strongly seems to help the elderly avoid dropping objects as often as they otherwise would.

However, that strategy could lead to reduced dexterity when older people are handling objects that require fine coordination. Or it could lead to premature fatigue of muscles when larger objects are lifted. At the same time, the elderly show relatively intact abilities to anticipate during manipulations that require their grasps to be simplified. When performing tasks of increasing complexity, however, age-related changes in anticipation begin to emerge. Thus, the relationships between the complexities of tasks and the degree of age-related changes suggest that results from simple and controlled laboratory experiments can only partially explain the impairments observed in more complex activities. This is true because most laboratory-based tasks have been limited to the grasping and handling of objects when the elderly are seated. Such experiments also focus on just one task and often eliminate the consequences of gravity and/or behavior.

In daily living, gravity is always present and there are behavioral consequences of the unsuccessful grasping and moving of objects. Moreover, the control of one's grip involves the coordination of multiple body parts that occurs simultaneously with other cognitive or motor tasks. Hence, future experiments should include tasks like the handling of fluid-filled containers and/or carrying objects while talking or walking. Such tasks, which have been investigated in healthy young people, are important because they are dynamic, involve the coordination of multiple physiological components (for example, changes in the forces of inertia are induced by whole-body movement), include periodic adjustments in one's grasp, and require the partitioning of attention between walking and grasping. Among other things, the aims of such experiments would be to maintain or restore manual dexterity to a level that is suitable to the activities of daily living among the elderly.

On June 23, 2013, while I was writing this chapter, Nik Wallenda, the thirty-four-year-old seventh-generation member of the famous Flying Wallendas, successfully walked across a tributary of the Grand Canyon on a two-inch-thick wire cable and holding a long pole to help balance himself. The rim-to-rim distance of 1,400 feet (a little more than a quarter mile) took him twenty-three minutes to complete (a velocity of about one foot per second). The cable was suspended 1,500 feet above the Little Colorado River, on Navajo Nation territory, because authorities at the Grand Canyon National Park would not grant the permission needed to achieve the feat in a more prominent sector of the Grand Canyon. Wallenda said he had been worried about only one thing, the gusts of wind that rise unpredictably from the canyon floor. Not long before the stunt was initiated, a gust of forty-eight miles per hour was recorded near the site. To compensate, Wallenda said he prayed nearly constantly as he walked. About fifteen minutes into the attempt, he had to stop and sit down on the wire because of its increasing motion and instability. At that point he said he felt like calling out "Mommy!" and not getting up.

Wallenda's accomplishment was noteworthy for many reasons, two of which were the lack of a safety harness and the absence of netting to break a potential fall. Arguably, Wallenda was at the peak of his musculoskeletal conditioning at the time of this daredevil stunt. His proprioception (interactions between the central and peripheral nervous systems and corresponding joints and muscles—that is, the ability to sense and maintain one's body position in space taking into account time and other conditions) and his sensorimotor and musculoskeletal functions had to be in near-perfect physiological condition. After this record-setting event, Wallenda said he hopes his next tight-wire achievement will be walking between the Chrysler and Empire State Buildings in New York City. Few if any entertainers possess the strength, balance, and endurance to perform such stunts in old age.

Aging and the Development and Function of Mitochondria

Of the many physiological parameters affected by aging, the malfunction and decreased development of mitochondria exert some of the most damaging effects. As the synthesis of new mitochondria decreases with age, the replacement of aging mitochondria and their contents is slower, which leads to the accumulation of modified lipids, proteins, and damaged DNA. This further aggravates problems with mitochondrial biochemistry and physiology.

The precise mechanism(s) behind the decrease in synthesis of mitochondria with age is unknown. However, it seems that both extra- and intracellular regulatory factors are involved. For example, subcellular signaling of mitochondria, including the synthesis and turnover of important regulatory molecules and their diffusion to the cytosol, is modified and thus contributes to the reduced development of mitochondria in older animals. If this is true of signaling molecules such as nitric oxide and hydrogen peroxide, then it must also be true for other molecules such as superoxide anion, peroxynitrite, and hydroxyl radical (to name just a few). The latter are damaging oxidants that have deleterious effects on tissues at any age.

Among the known intracellular regulators of mitochondrial development, the enzymatic activity of adenine monophosphate kinase (AMPK), the so-called fuel or energy gauge of the mammalian muscle cell, appears to be one of the main factors associated with mitochondrial malfunction, insulin resistance, and impaired lipid metabolism in aging cells. AMPK is positioned at a critical cellular-molecular junction in a complex signaling network that integrates metabolism and aging. It plays critical roles in processes such as control of insulin resistance, obesity, oxidation of fatty acids, and development and function of mitochondria. Therefore, its dysfunction seems to be a key element in mitochondrial activity and regulation of metabolism during aging.

Chronic inactivation of AMPK is linked to decreased synthesis and development of mitochondria in aged animals. Moreover, reduced activity of AMPK correlates with aging-related resistance to insulin and to the insufficient use of intracellular fat. The converse is also true. In *Caenorhabditis elegans*, a worm-like invertebrate, overexpression of aak-2, the animal's equivalent of AMPK, resulted in an increase in longevity. Because of findings like these and the near-universal distribution of AMPK in the animal kingdom, scientists believe that chronic activation of AMPK might be a way to slow aging. Additional anti-aging strategies that could reduce mitochondrial dysfunction are also being considered. For example, researchers have observed that supplementing the diet with vitamin E (and/or other antioxidant vitamins such as A and C) and performing moderate physical activity reduce mitochondrial dysfunction in the elderly. In addition, reduced intake of calories and increased physical activity have been shown to increase the activity of several key enzymes and to enhance the synthesis and development of mitochondria.

Restriction of calories affects some of the main factors involved in mitochondrial function, leading to increased concentrations of nitric oxide. However, it is not clear if long-term restriction of calories affects the long-term function of AMPK, even if short-term restriction in calories increases the phosphorylation and thereby the activity of AMPK in both young and old animals. In *C. elegans*, restricting the intake of energy bypasses the need for aak-2 activity to extend the life span. However, it is not clear if restricting the intake of energy affects mitochondrial synthesis in all tissues, or if its effects are specific to selected cells and tissues. It also seems that restricting calories affects mitochondrial activities in the skeletal muscle of aged animals but not in young ones.

The decline in oxidative capacity in type I and IIa skeletal muscle fibers in aging is attenuated by the restriction of calories in older animals. It has been suggested that the age-dependent decline in mitochondrial function in both human cardiac and skeletal muscle can be improved with restricted intake of calories. Investigators have recently reported that resveratrol, a polyphenol, affects the synthesis and development of mitochondria in the liver, muscle, and brain, and that these actions are explained by resveratrol's ability to activate sirtuins, which are known to be promoters of mitochondrial and cellular health. The actions of resveratrol are lost in mice that have had the responsible sirtuin gene knocked out. Resveratrol is also able to increase the activity of AMPK and the life span of *C. elegans* that overexpress sirtuins.

Resveratrol not only maintains mitochondrial development and health, but it also affects other aging-related processes such as insulin resistance and the metabolism of lipids. Reducing the intake of calories and administering resveratrol modify mitochondrial activity by switching the mitochondria's source of energy from glucose to fatty acids. In the case of diet, this happens because both fasting and reducing intake of calories simultaneously enhance the breakdown and inhibit the synthesis of fatty acids. For example, inhibiting the enzyme fatty acid synthase in the hypothalamus increases the number of mitochondria in skeletal muscle by increasing the levels of malonyl-CoA. The malonyl-CoA signal is transmitted by the sympathetic nervous system to skeletal muscle, where it increases the oxidation of fatty acids and the expenditure of energy from lipids.

Some of the beneficial effects mediated by reducing one's intake of calories, having low levels of stress, and/or engaging in regular moderate exercise have been associated with hormesis. Hormesis is one term used to express the generally favorable physiological responses to reduced exposures to toxins and other stressors. Hormetic responses trigger protective and reparative reactions, including mitochondrial synthesis and a higher turnover of aging and impaired subcellular organelles. Hormesis has been suggested to explain the effects of exercise on mitochondrial activity and development in muscle. If true, this would imply that the beneficial effects of exercise on mitochondrial synthesis and development are independent of age.

The Role of Mitochondrial Fission and Fusion in Aging

Another concept related to the activity of mitochondria during aging is mitochondrial fission and fusion. Mitochondrial fusion means that two immature, undeveloped mitochondria come together to form a single mitochondrion. Mitochondrial fission, on the other hand, describes the division of a single mitochondrion into two components. Both are integral to the homeostasis of mitochondrial development, maturation, and aging. Mitochondria are dynamic organelles (mitodynamics) with complex mechanisms for fusion and fission. These processes ensure mitochondrial remodeling and allow morphological transitions from individual, subcellular structures to complex cellular networks such as scaffolding and tubules. All this is regulated by proteins whose physiological functions are critical to mitochondrial activity, and whose dysfunction is associated with pathophysiological states such as Alzheimer's and Parkinson's diseases. Activity of these proteins and their associated genes is essential for the maintenance of mitochondrial DNA, as has been demonstrated in yeast. More recently, the mitochondrial fission-related protein fis-1 has been associated with improved aging in mammalian cell cultures (see below).

As the last few pages of this chapter reveal, mitochondria play a central role in the aging process. This is especially true in large organs that contribute significantly to total body mass (for example, skeletal muscle, skin, liver, and brain). In these organs, each cell might possess several hundred to a thousand mitochondria. Each mitochondrion has eight to twelve copies of mitochondrial DNA, but this number diminishes with aging and cellular damage. Ultimately, in elderly individuals these losses show up as diminutions in many physiological functions such as walking and getting around, manipulating objects, hearing and seeing. For example, depletion of fis-1 induced swelling and flattening of the organelle and reduced electron density. Such changes have been correlated with impaired growth of cells, a marker of aging. Restoration of the concentrations of fis-1 restored the growth of cells, confirming that fis-1 plays an important role in cellular aging.

Additionally, sustained elongation of mitochondria was linked to decreased electrical properties of the mitochondrial double membrane, increased generation of reactive oxygen species, and damage to DNA. Thus, it is becoming increasingly clear that both the morphology and physiology of mitochondria are important elements in cellular aging and dysfunction. For this reason, the physiology and pathophysiology of the mitochondria during aging, in conjunction with the genes and proteins that regulate mitochondrial function, merit further investigation.

Maintenance of mitochondrial development and function during aging is crucial to minimizing or preventing the progression of age-related diseases that affect muscle and other organs or systems. Adopting and maintaining a healthy lifestyle that includes regular, moderate physical activity is good for healthy aging. So is a low-calorie diet including copious quantities of grains, vegetables, and fruits; the prudent consumption of meat; and few or no large, sugary soft drinks, fruit juices, alcohol, tea, and coffee (as a rule water will do). Supplementing this kind of diet and physical activity with frequent social outlets seems to be another way to achieve mitochondrial health and cellular viability during aging.

With people sixty years of age and older representing the fastest-growing fraction of the global population, there will continue to be a corresponding increase in the prevalence of limitations in mobility. To minimize these aging-related limitations, encouragement from family, friends, neighbors, and health care providers—will be necessary but not sufficient. What will also be needed is an increasing knowledge of the physiological mechanisms that impair mobility and physical function as we age. An additional benefit of acquiring this physiological information will be our ability to develop therapeutic interventions to assist the elderly in maintaining their independence throughout life.

I and thousands like me have practiced healthy living (diet, exercise, and avoiding harmful substances such as alcohol and tobacco) for many years. Perhaps future magic bullets will come in the form of drugs, nutriceuticals, and other agents, but until then this (diet, exercise, and avoidance of harmful substances) is a successful formula for living a long, active, healthy life. Consider, for example, the world's Senior Olympians, many of whom are still competing at ages of seventy-five to a hundred years. If you would like further evidence, then also consider the thousands of Mormons who, among many other positive lifestyle choices, follow the Word of Wisdom, discussed in chapter I. These men and women have enjoyed the rewards of the Mormon lifestyle for decades and outlive the general population by eight to ten years.

9

The Aging Cardiovascular System

The Organization and Function of the Cardiovascular System

Arguably, the cardiovascular system can be reduced to two organs and a tissue: the heart, the blood vessels, and the circulating blood. Blood is considered a tissue but not an organ because it is composed of cellular elements, as are all tissues (for example, red blood cells, white blood cells) that are suspended in an aqueous extracellular matrix, the plasma. During development of the human zygote and its first two successors—the conceptus and embryo—in the uterus, all three components of the cardiovascular system develop concurrently. The maturation of the embryonic heart is called cardiogenesis. A beat in the neonatal heart can be detected as early as eighteen to twenty-one days after conception. The development of the blood vessels is referred to as angiogenesis, and the synthesis of blood cells is called erythropoiesis (for red blood cells only) or hematopoiesis (for all blood cells and noncellular elements in the blood).

The detailed, underlying physiological mechanisms of the concurrent growth and development of these three components of the cardiovascular system is a mystery that surpasses current human understanding. But think of the downstream miracle: just when the delivery of oxygen and nutrients to the developing conceptus and embryo is approaching the physical limits of diffusion, a cardiovascular system appears on the scene. The two new entities (embryo and cardiovascular system) then mature in parallel. Logically, there would be no need for a pump (the heart) if it could not circulate something somewhere. What the pump circulates—the blood cells, the plasma, and all the other elements—would also be pointless if a system of channels was not available to contain and direct the flow of blood (the blood vessels). The development of our marvelous bodies is laden with brilliant examples of near-perfect organization, purpose, and timing.

Many details about the human cardiovascular system are not appropriate for this book. However, some additional information will help clarify the effects of aging on this system. The healthy, fully developed human heart has four chambers, whose functions include: to separate more-oxygenated from less-oxygenated blood, to develop greater and lesser pressure gradients between two locations, and to eject blood into two vascular systems that lie in series one with another (the pulmonary and systemic circulatory systems).

The aorta delivers blood from the left ventricle of the heart to the systemic circulatory system. The corresponding pulmonary artery simultaneously delivers blood from the right ventricle of the heart to the pulmonary circulatory system. In both cases, a similar volume of blood (for example, seventy-five milliliters)—called the stroke volume—passes, sequentially, through large arteries, small arteries, and arterioles, ultimately entering the smallest blood vessels, the capillaries. Capillaries are the vessel segments where most of the exchange between the blood and surrounding tissues takes place—for example, oxygen and glucose are delivered to the tissues, and carbon dioxide and other byproducts are released from the tissues. Capillary blood, with its chemistry that is significantly different from upstream arteriolar blood, is then passed on sequentially, to the venules, small veins, and large veins, and ultimately reaches the right atrium, the anatomical end of the systemic circulatory system.

The blood that fills the right atrium is called a venous admixture. This phrase derives from the fact that venous blood coming from each of the many organs and tissues served by the systemic circulatory system varies in chemical composition. Thus, venous blood of differing chemical compositions gets mixed inside the right atrium. The venous admixture is then passed into the right ventricle and subsequently ejected, sequentially, into the pulmonary artery, pulmonary circulatory system, and lungs. In the lungs another exchange takes place. Carbon dioxide and other waste gases are exhausted to the ambient air, and atmospheric oxygen is simultaneously delivered to the pulmonary capillaries. The pulmonary capillary blood is then delivered sequentially to the left atrium (which marks the end of the pulmonary circulatory system), the left ventricle, and the systemic circulatory system (via the aorta). That completes the circuit.

The above text describes, in simple terms, the organization of the cardiovascular system in all mammals, not just humans. Of course there are subtle differences across the species, but the same general organization and function is common to them all. The cardiovascular system is the first mammalian organ system to complete its functional development embryologically. From the above discussion one can understand the reason for this. Because it develops earlier, one could also argue that the cardiovascular system begins to age earlier. Nonetheless, the cardiovascular system is designed, I believe, to function for a minimum of about 120 years (see the discussion of supercentenarians in chapter 1). Of course through neglect (such as poor diet and abuse of drugs or alcohol), disuse (sedentary lifestyles), congenital disorders, accidents, and the like, some cardiovascular systems and their caretakers live for much shorter periods of time (for example, the actor James Gandolfini died of a heart attack and cardiac arrest in June 2013, at the age of fifty-one).

Anemia and the Cardiovascular System

The most abundant cellular element in human whole blood is the red blood cell. In the typical healthy American adult, there are 4.5–5.5 million red blood cells in each microliter of whole blood. The next most abundant cellular element is the blood platelet (which is actually a cellular fragment, since it lacks a nucleus). The least abundant cellular element is the white blood cell. Other defining characteristics of whole blood are the hematocrit, the hemoglobin content, the contents and/or partial pressures of important blood gases such as oxygen and carbon dioxide, and the electrolytes. Each of these has well-defined limits in the healthy young adult that can change markedly with age.

Collectively, the above and other distinguishing characteristics of the blood can rightfully be called blood chemistry, which is one of the foundations of internal medicine. Knowing one's blood chemistry is prudent. Such knowledge can be achieved only by seeing your physician for annual or biannual visits that include the collection of venous blood samples and having them exposed to clinical analyzers and other instruments for analysis. Obtaining and then retaining copies of these reports are the patient's obligation, opportunity, and right. I strongly encourage the reader to begin such a practice. It will pay long-term dividends.

While editing the last chapters of this book, I had my most recent physician's physical examination. It included a comprehensive blood evaluation. I was not surprised by the results. For example, my blood sugar (92 milligrams per deciliter of whole blood [mgdL]) and cholesterol (177 mg/dL) were both elevated. Typically these values range from 75–80 and 125–50, respectively, in my blood. I was annoyed, but I understood the changes. I had been fasting as my doctor instructed when the blood was withdrawn, but for the two or three weeks before that exam, my wife and I had been entertaining out-of-town guests. We did many things with them that could be described as eating poorly. For example, we all indulged in an excess of sweets and fatty foods in restaurants. This took the place of our usual homemade meals that routinely include vegetables, fruits, and other healthier choices. That same blood chemistry report found my platelets to be low, but warning signs of anemia (low hematocrit, low red blood cell count, and so on) and other markers of healthy whole blood were normal.

One of the warning signs of cardiovascular aging is anemia, or low circulating content of red blood cells. Anemia correlates with aging-related conditions such as cancer, diabetes, hypertension, and other cardiovascular diseases, but it is often ignored. If anemia is mild, it might be considered of lesser importance than other conditions that carry a higher rate of mortality. Furthermore, there are no research-based guidelines for the diagnosis and treatment of anemia in the elderly, which makes it difficult for the physician to choose a course of action. Epidemiological studies link anemia with morbidity and mortality in older adults, but these studies have yet to be followed by clinical trials showing that anemia is significantly correlated with the loss of functional ability and survival of the elderly. Additionally, there are large gaps in our knowledge of the impact of aging on hematopoiesis and erythropoiesis.

The World Health Organization defines anemia as a hemoglobin concentration less than twelve grams per deciliter for women (<12.0 gm/dL) and thirteen grams per deciliter (<13.0 gm/dL) for men, a definition that has stood for nearly fifty years. Data from the World Health Organization indicate that anemia affects about 10 percent of people over age sixty-five around the world, and that the incidence increases to 20 percent in adults over age eighty-five. Anemia is also significantly correlated with mortality in older adults and with cognitive, functional, and physical decline. Despite high-quality biochemical data, a large percentage of cases of the disease in older adults is not attributable to any clear cause and is therefore called unexplained anemia of the elderly.

Anemia and erythropoietin are intricately related. Erythropoietin is the primary physiological factor that promotes the survival of stem cell precursors and their transformation into red blood cells. Erythropoietin is a central regulator of erythropoiesis, and circulating erythropoietin is tightly regulated by the kidney and other organs. For example, when the quantity of oxygen in the blood decreases (hypoxia), the kidneys release more erythropoietin. This promotes greater production and release of red blood cells from bone marrow. The increased number of red blood cells compensates for the low oxygen by increasing the blood's capacity to carry oxygen.

Circulating concentrations of erythropoietin have been shown to increase with age in people with a hemoglobin concentration greater than or equal to 14.0 gm/dL. This suggests that the efficiency of erythropoietin signaling declines with age. There is considerable agreement among researchers that concentrations of erythropoietin are low in unexplained anemia of the elderly, when compared to iron-deficiency anemia. However, the release of erythropoietin seems to be uniquely sensitive to iron deficiency, and this is probably due to the requirement of iron for enzymes that degrade hypoxia-inducible factor, a critical molecular transcription factor required for expression and release of erythropoietin.

People who suffer from unexplained anemia of the elderly display features of inflammation. A subclinical, pro-inflammatory state independent of disease is widely accepted as one of the basic biological processes underlying aging. Though the physiological mechanisms underlying age-related inflammation are unclear, it is known that the accumulation of reactive oxygen species activates molecular factors that induce the release of numerous pro-inflammatory chemicals. The inflammation of aging is more qualitative than quantitative and has been inferred from laboratory tests such as the erythrocyte (red blood cell) sedimentation rate and C-reactive protein. The concentrations of C-reactive protein in the plasma have been used as markers for low-grade inflammation in the development of clinical trials for the treatment of aging-related cardiovascular disease and diabetes. Other important mediators of inflammation used primarily for research include the pro-inflammatory chemicals interleukin-6, tumor necrosis factor alpha, and interferon gamma.

By being toxic to bone marrow, both prescription and nonprescription drugs can contribute to anemia in older patients. Alcohol, a drug, is probably the most common nonprescription offender. Chemotherapy, immunosuppressive drugs, drugs that inhibit folate metabolism, drugs against human immunodeficiency virus or other viral diseases, and radiation treatment all cause anemia. Moreover, most of these same treatments do injury to or in other ways harm the heart and blood vessels. Cancer-related chemotherapy and radiation are no exceptions. Thus, the combination of low oxygen-carrying capacity of the blood (anemia) and an injured cardiovascular system is a formula for unintended but unavoidable damage and potential death from medical therapy. Proving that a medication or treatment is causing anemia usually requires discontinuation of the drug, followed by careful observation and collection of several blood samples over time (weeks or months).

Decreased circulating concentrations of testosterone and other androgens have been associated with the development of anemia in older men and women, and specifically with unexplained anemia in the elderly. For several decades, scientists have known that androgens promote erythropoiesis, though the physiological mechanism involved has not been identified. Estrogen has also been shown to stimulate telomerase activity. Activity of the enzyme telomerase is a critical feature of all cells, but it is especially important in those with high replicative capacity such as hematopoietic stem cells and red blood cell progenitors. By inducing telomerase, estrogen is expected to maintain genetic homeostasis and therefore cellular viability. Additionally, hypothyroidism can cause anemia, but it is unknown if the mild increase in thyroid-stimulating hormone observed in aging contributes to unexplained anemia in the elderly.

Aging Red Blood Cells

During the last month of gestation and following birth, red blood cells are produced exclusively by the bone marrow. Before this the liver, spleen, and lymph tissue are the main sites of production of red blood cells. Until about five years of age, the marrow of all bones produces red blood cells. This production declines in the long bones until it stops completely at about age twenty. From that point on, the main sites of production of red blood cells are the ribs, the sternum, and the vertebrae. The proximal portions of long bones such as the humerus and tibia, as well as the pelvic girdle, also contribute to the production of red blood cells after age twenty.

Once delivered into the circulation from the marrow, red blood cells normally circulate for an average of 120 days. Even though mature red blood cells lack endoplasmic reticulum, mitochondria, and nuclei (sites of the production of proteins), they do have cytosolic enzymes that can metabolize glucose and produce small amounts of energy. These enzymes perform other tasks as well, such as preventing intracellular proteins from oxidation, maintaining transport mechanisms across cell membranes, sustaining the elasticity of the red cell membrane, and maintaining intracellular iron in the ferrous rather than the ferric state. The latter is necessary for the proper function of hemoglobin.

The aging of our bodies in general is caused by many things, including the wearing down of enzymatic metabolic processes. In addition, the repetitive deformation as the red blood cell recirculates through capillaries whose internal diameters are smaller than the external diameter of the cell causes cellular fragility. This leads to the rupture of the cell membranes, loss of hemoglobin, and termination of function. If this doesn't happen in the systemic and pulmonary capillaries, it does in the spleen, where the spaces through which the cells pass are only two or three micrometers in diameter, as opposed to the eight-micrometer diameter of the average red blood cell. When the membranes of the cells burst, the hemoglobin is phagocytized almost immediately by macrophages. After a few days of phagocytosis, the macrophages release iron back into the circulation. The recirculated iron is carried by a transport protein called transferrin to either the bone marrow for the production of new red blood cells or to the liver for storage as ferritin. Another portion of the phagocytized hemoglobin is converted to the bile pigment bilirubin, which is stored in the bile and used later in digestive processes.

The fragility of red blood cells, aging or otherwise, can be tested by placing them in saline solutions of varying strengths. The plasma that these cells normally circulate in has a salinity of 0.9 percent. The osmotic pressure of this salt concentration makes it isotonic (also isosmotic) with the cytoplasm inside the red blood cell. Therefore, in 0.9 percent saline red blood cells remain intact: they do not rupture. If the strength of the salt solution is increased, say to 1.8 percent, the red blood cell loses intracellular water and shrinks. If the solution is reduced to 0.5 percent, water is drawn into the cell, and it begins to swell. When the solution is reduced further, say to 0.45 percent, the cell will burst (hemolyze). Hemolysis (the process by which the cell releases its hemoglobin into the solution) is complete when the salt solution decreases to 0.35 percent.

If one collects a sample of either venous or arterial whole blood in a test tube, the fraction of that sample (in other words, following centrifugation) that is composed of cellular elements, including mainly red blood cells, is the hematocrit. In healthy young adult males the fraction is about 45 percent. The balance of the volume, 55 percent, is plasma. In healthy young women the corresponding number for hematocrit is closer to 40 percent. The difference is caused by the loss of blood during a woman's monthly menstrual cycle. During the years or decades after menopause, depending on a woman's state of health, her hematocrit might rise a few percent to 42–43 percent.

The most important protein inside each healthy red blood cell is hemoglobin. Hemoglobin molecules are suspended in intracellular cytoplasm and are concentrated around the perimeter of the red blood cell, a biconcave disk-like cell. The biconcavity of the red blood cell increases the ratio of surface area to cell volume. This maximizes the surface area for the diffusion of oxygen into and carbon dioxide out of the cell. The density of hemoglobin molecules at the inside perimeter of the cell reduces the distance that oxygen has to diffuse from the plasma to hemoglobin. Each of these qualities—that is, membrane surface area, high ratio of surface area to volume, and diffusion distance for respiratory gases— enhances the exchange of blood gases between intra- and extracellular spaces.

In the human adult, hemoglobin is a polypeptide composed of two alpha and two beta chains of amino acids. It is often designated HbA for adult hemoglobin (as opposed to HbF for fetal hemoglobin and HbS for sickle cell hemoglobin). When healthy and whole, each molecule of HbA can carry four molecules of oxygen. This amounts to about 1.34 mL of molecular oxygen for each gram of hemoglobin. In healthy young adults there are about 13–15 grams of HbA in each 100 mL of whole blood (more in men than in women). This means that when all of the molecules of HbA in each gram of HbA are fully saturated with molecular oxygen, each 100 mL of whole blood can carry about 17–20 mL of oxygen. This is called the oxygen-carrying capacity. When breathing atmospheric oxygen at sea level, a healthy young adult will have 98–99 percent of his or her hemoglobin molecules saturated with molecular oxygen. These numbers are important, as they help guide physicians when caring for the sick and injured. They also help inform experimental physiologists about the respiratory status of tissues, organs, and whole animals. And, for the purposes of this subsection, they help describe the effects of aging on the cardiovascular system.

Since the beginning of the twenty-first century, anemia has emerged as a risk factor for a variety of adverse outcomes in older adults, including hospitalization, disability, and mortality. Physiologically, anemia is a homeostatic imbalance in the circulating concentrations of hemoglobin wherein the production of red blood cells is exceeded by their rates of destruction. According to epidemiological data, the prevalence of anemia among both men and women ages sixty years and older is about 10 percent. The majority of cases are mild, with less than 1–3 percent of older adults who live in the community (that is, who are not in an institution such as a nursing home) having hemoglobin concentrations <10–11 gm/dL. The prevalence of anemia in men is lowest between ages seventeen and forty-nine years, while for women anemia is least common at ages fifty to sixty-four years. In women this argues for a partial reversal of the condition in the postmenopausal state. At ages seventy-five to eighty-four years researchers have estimated that as many as 15 percent of men and as few as 7 percent of women are anemic (another bit of evidence of postmenopausal improvement in women). In people eighty-five years and older, anemia was present in 30 percent of men and only 17 percent of women.

The crossover effect (in this case, the epidemiological conclusions that men are more likely to have anemia at older ages, while women are more likely to have it at younger ages) reflects the application of gender-specific criteria for defining anemia. For example, in the case of the World Health Organization's criteria, men with hemoglobin concentrations of 12.0–12.9 gm/dL are considered anemic, but women with these concentrations are considered normal. If women with these concentrations were considered anemic, the prevalence of anemia in women ages sixty-five years and older would rise to 33 percent. Furthermore, the prevalence in women ages sixty-five to seventy-four would be 30 percent; in women seventy-five to eighty-four, 35 percent; and in women older than eighty-five, 43 percent. Under these conditions, the overall prevalence of anemia in older adults would double, to 23 percent. Thus, more epidemiological research is needed to define the hemoglobin concentrations below which the risk of adverse effects is increased in older men and women.

In addition to differences in gender, there are marked differences in race when it comes to hemoglobin. As early as the 1930s, investigators observed that blacks have lower hemoglobin concentrations than whites do. Such differences are not explained by health, nutrition, or socioeconomic status and are observed at all ages, including in healthy children and younger adults. Indeed, it is not surprising that the incidence of anemia is two to three times higher in blacks than in whites when the World Health Organization's criteria are applied. It is plausible that genetic mutations selected by different environmental pressures in Africa and Europe contribute to racial differences in hemoglobin concentrations. For example, thalassemia and deficiency of the enzyme glucose-6-phosphatase are inborn errors of metabolism in red blood cells. They are known to confer survival benefits from malarial infections and are more common in blacks than in whites. One study showed that racial differences in hemoglobin concentration narrowed after excluding African American participants with iron deficiency, thalassemia, and sickle cell traits. However, differences in hemoglobin concentrations remained significant, suggesting that unidentified adaptive factors likely exist. One study found that the prevalence of anemia (as defined by the World Health Organization) in the United States was about 9 percent in older non-Hispanic white men and women, but in older non-Hispanic black men and women it was about

28 percent. The distribution of hemoglobin concentrations among older Mexican American men and women is about 10 percent.

Aside from changes in hemoglobin concentrations with time, individual molecules undergo aging-related changes in structure and function. In the case of hemoglobin, as each molecule of oxygen binds to the hemoglobin molecule, conformational changes in the protein occur. These changes affect the ease or difficulty with which subsequent molecules of oxygen bind, making it easier or harder for the second and third than for the first and fourth molecules. The relationship is illustrated graphically by the oxyhemoglobin saturation curve. This curve describes the influence of partial pressures of oxygen that is dissolved in plasma (the independent variable) on the binding of molecular oxygen to hemoglobin (the dependent variable). The reader can learn more about this physiological relationship by consulting any good textbook on physiology.

Oxidative stress in red blood cells plays an important role in the pathogenesis of anemia in patients with beta thalassemia (a condition in which beta chains of hemoglobin molecules develop improperly). Elevated oxidative stress accelerates aging, increases the rate of programmed cell death of erythrocytes, and shortens the life span of red blood cells. Exogenously administered antioxidants have been shown to reduce plasma-induced oxidative stress and to increase the numbers of circulating red blood cells in patients suffering from thalassemia. Thus, antioxidants reduce the severity of anemia in these patients by inhibiting the efflux of glutathione, a naturally occurring antioxidant that is found in most cells, including erythrocytes (that is, the summation of exogenous plus endogenous antioxidants increases the total antioxidant pool). Also, oxidant overload and the subsequent cellular stress it causes accelerate aging, increase the rate of programmed cell death, and shorten the life span of erythrocytes. Investigators have found that challenging red blood cells with hydrogen peroxide causes a decrease in intracellular glutathione and a corresponding increase in the efflux of glutathione. It has also been shown that circulating red blood cells from patients with thalassemia have lower oxidized and total glutathione concentrations. In addition, the oxidative challenge has been demonstrated to induce glutathione efflux from erythrocytes of healthy subjects. Oxidative stress is considered a central player in the pathogenesis of anemia.

The Aging Heart

The aging heart undergoes functional, structural, and molecular changes. Functional changes include decreased left ventricular diastolic compliance, impaired relaxation during diastole, reduced early diastolic filling, increased late diastolic filling, impaired left ventricular ejection and heart rate reserve, altered heart rhythm and increased cardiac arrhythmias, deficits in sympathetic and parasympathetic regulation of heart rate and left ventricular contractility, prolongation of cardiac action potentials, changes in the coronary vasculature and coronary blood flow, increased pulse pressure, and endothelial dysfunction. There are more changes, but time and space preclude a detailed discussion.

Structural changes occur at the tissue and cellular levels. These include increased left ventricular wall thickness, decrease in total number of cardiomyocytes (increased apoptosis and necrosis), increased size of myocytes (myocyte hypertrophy), increased content of collagen in connective tissue, increased cardiac fibrosis, decreased number of pacemaker cells, reduced number of cardiac stem cells, and increased thickness of the walls of the aorta and coronary vessels. The latter characteristic is often difficult to distinguish from the effects of age-related diseases (for example, arteriosclerosis).

At the molecular level, aging-induced changes include attenuated responses to stimulation of cardiac nerves, decreased numbers of cardiac receptors, impaired homeostasis of calcium ions (for example, impaired pumping of calcium by intracellular organelles), reduced genetic expression and activity of proteins that make calcium pumps, impaired mitochondrial function (such as accumulated mutations and deletions within mitochondrial DNA), loss of mitochondria, increased accumulation of oxidative damage, alterations in cardiac metabolism, decrease in oxidation and use of fat by the myocardium, impairments in the renin-angiotensin-aldosterone system (although this is more a kidney problem, even though concentrations of cardiac angiotensin II increase with age), and reduced signaling by insulin and insulin-like growth factors.

The above age-related changes in the heart can occur even when no contributing cardiac risk factors such as hypertension or diabetes exist. Due to apoptosis, necrosis, and autophagy (self-destruction), these changes lead to a 35 percent loss of cardiac myocytes, accompanied by a 20 percent decrease in pacemaker cells in the sinoatrial node. As defined by the expression of markers of cellular aging and the occurrence of shorter telomeres, the aging heart also contains more aged cardiac myofibers. The time-dependent loss of healthy cardiomyocytes is accompanied by a marked decline in regenerative capacity from 1 percent per year at age twenty to less than half of this at age seventy-five.

Age-related left ventricular changes can include hypertrophy and failure of diastolic function, resulting in elevated end diastolic pressure. An elevation in this pressure can impede the return of pulmonary venous blood to the left ventricle and can result in pulmonary congestion. This, in turn, can cause impaired respiratory function, including the exchange of blood gases. The cumulative effect of these and related changes, accompanied by other diseases, can predispose older people to develop diastolic heart failure. This is defined as the symptoms of heart failure with physiological systolic but impaired diastolic function, atrial fibrillation, and cardiac ischemia.

Cardiac myocytes possess an unusually high density of mitochondria due to their extraordinary demand for energy in the form of ATP. The mitochondrion is the main cellular location of glycolysis (use of stored glycogen for energy), oxidative phosphorylation, and other biochemical processes (for example, the oxidation of fatty acids) that are involved in the production of ATP and other energy sources. Except for several subunits of the chain of oxidative phosphorylation that are encoded by mitochondrial genes, most mitochondrial proteins are encoded by the nucleus. Therefore, the development of mitochondria is regulated at the genetic level by a set of nuclear coactivators and transcription factors. The first of these was identified in brown adipose tissue. Subsequently, two more related coactivators were identified. Each of these coactivators has been demonstrated to coordinate mitochondrial development and function through association with related transcription factors. The coactivators and transcription factors drive the expression of mitochondrial genes that are important in the production of mitochondrial energy, the generation of ATP, and the maintenance of cardiac function.

Changes in the aging mitochondria include increased reactive oxygen species, impaired oxidative phosphorylation, reduced synthesis of ATP,

failure in the oxidation of fatty acids, and increased mutations in mitochondrial DNA. The physiological relevance of such alterations in the
aging cardiovascular system, and in the heart in particular, has been documented in patients with genetic disorders. People in whom congenital
and aging-related mutations lead to loss of function in genes essential for
the development of mitochondrial DNA, oxidation of fatty acids, and
oxidative phosphorylation develop enlarged hearts and the cardiovascular
impediments that accompany them. Examples include disturbances in the
regulation of blood volume, blood flow, and blood pressure. In addition,
congestive heart failure and edema and inflammation of the limbs and
other peripheral organs and tissues are common in cases of enlarged,
failing hearts.

Although mutations of a single gene highlight the importance of a
specific process in the physiology of cardiac function, there are often compromises of multiple mitochondrial processes in the aging heart. This is
due, at least in part, to increasing concentrations of reactive oxygen
and nitrogen species in the mitochondria. Increased reactive oxygen and
nitrogen species in the mitochondria leads to increasing damage to
mitochondrial DNA, elements of the electron transport chain, and
other mitochondrial structures and functions, and this is consistent with
the mitochondrial–free radical theory of aging. In animal experiments,
investigators have found that overexpressing the antioxidant enzyme
mitochondrial catalase reduces damage to proteins and to mitochondrial
DNA, prevents functional decline in the heart, and increases median life
span. Overexpression of mitochondrial catalase also reduces the oxidant-
induced enlargement of the heart observed in mice.

In our laboratory, my colleagues and I have found impressive mitochondrial protective actions for acetaminophen. Acetaminophen is the
active ingredient in many over-the-counter analgesics and pain relievers.
We have observed acetaminophen-mediated protection in the hearts of
guinea pigs and dogs, and in the brains of rats and mice. For example,
when these organs are exposed to tissue damage caused by ischemia and
reperfusion, hypoxia and reoxygenation, or exogenously administered oxidants like peroxynitrite, the mitochondria are swollen and electron sparse
(very light). Under physiological conditions, mitochondria from the heart
and brain are unswollen, appear ellipsoidal, and are electron dense (very

dark). In hearts, the symmetrical arrangement of muscle filaments is disrupted by ischemia and reperfusion and protected by acetaminophen.

Corresponding cellular or molecular evidence of damage in our experiments is the increased appearance of cytochrome C in the intracellular fluid during ischemia, hypoxia, and oxidant overload. Normally, cytochrome C remains inside the mitochondria. Acetaminophen minimizes the injury-induced translocation of cytochrome C. Additionally, one of the proteins that regulates movements of protons (such as the hydrogen ions that influence pH in cellular and extracellular fluids), the so-called mitochondrial permeability transition pore, is damaged by the above injuries, whereas it is not in the presence of acetaminophen.

Other specific targets of damaged mitochondrial DNA are complexes I and IV of the electron transport chain. Malfunctioning of these components of biochemical respiration leads to the reduced production of ATP; impairment of its role in activities such as excitation-contraction coupling; and development of enlarged, weakened hearts. Natural decline in activity of the electron transport chain has been noted in aged hearts in both humans and rodents. Other age-dependent changes in mitochondrial energy pathways that have been reported include decreased rates of oxidation of fatty acids and increased glycolysis in animal experiments on cardiac hypertrophy and heart failure.

Dysfunction of telomeres in the aging cardiovascular system of humans is another area of investigation that is just beginning to blossom. A causal role for telomere dysfunction in the aging and/or diseased human cardiovascular system is supported by several lines of evidence. First, clinical case reports indicate that cardiovascular disease might be more common in patients with gene mutations of the enzyme telomerase than was previously appreciated. Two members of the same family with dominant mutations in telomerase activity developed cardiac disease at an early age (an enlarged heart and severe cardiac fibrosis). In a separate case, a heart attack (myocardial infarction) at a young age was documented in a patient with mutated telomerase.

Other conditions involving impaired maintenance of telomeres (for example, Werner syndrome) are associated with premature cardiovascular disease. These include atherosclerosis, aortic stenosis, valvular disease, mitral regurgitation, and valvular and vascular calcification. Although experimental mice develop cardiac fibrosis of the Werner syndrome type, there are few cases of this condition in humans. For example, a seventeen-year-old with Werner syndrome has been identified. These reports might be intriguing, but systematic investigations of patients without symptoms are needed for precise quantification of the disorders.

Second, human cardiac muscle fibers and cardiac stem cells display an age-dependent decline in length of telomeres. They also express markers of aging. Such markers are consistent with the reduced proliferative and regenerative capacity of aging cardiac myocytes and cardiac stem cells. In cases of human heart failure, cardiomyocytes contain telomeres that are 25 percent shorter than those observed in age-matched healthy subjects. Consistent with this delongation of telomeres, there is a corresponding activation of enzymes to clear damaged DNA and increased apoptosis of cardiomyocytes.

And third, the relevance of critically short telomeres to the aging human heart is inferred from epidemiological studies that demonstrate associations between shortened telomeres, aging, and cardiovascular disease. In those studies, the lengths of telomeres in white blood cells were inversely related to multiple cardiovascular risk factors, including smoking, obesity, diabetes, systemic inflammation, and physical inactivity. In clinical studies, the decreased length of telomeres in white blood cells has been associated with coronary artery disease, premature myocardial infarction, coronary calcification, and increased thickness of the media of carotid arteries.

Another sign of the aging human heart is the appearance of cardiac arrhythmias. An arrhythmia is any disturbance of the physiological origination and/or conduction of cardiac action potentials that began in the sinoatrial node. Arrhythmias can range from the innocuous (for example, minor prolongations of the P-R interval in an electrocardiogram, or ventricular premature beats) to the potentially life threatening (such as sustained ventricular tachycardia and ventricular fibrillation). Many arrhythmias increase in both frequency and intensity with age. Some arrhythmias result from aging-related deterioration of the specialized conduction system. Others are caused by medications that the elderly are more likely than younger people to take. Still other arrhythmias result from negligence, such as being physically inactive, being overweight or obese, and having a nutritionally poor diet. Finally, chemo- and radiation treatment are known causes of damage to the otherwise healthy heart.

With aging, the incidence of cardiac arrhythmias increases at rest and during exercise. Also, a marked reduction in the number of cells that constitute the sinoatrial node is observed with age. The reduction is usually caused by apoptosis and can result in less than 10 percent of the mass of pacemaker cells remaining by age seventy. However, this is not as alarming as it may sound, because it takes only one cell to serve as the cardiac pacemaker. If the pacemaker cell wears out, others are ready to take its place. In healthy aging, pacemaker cells in the human heart are a sustainable resource. These slow-response, modified cardiac myocytes are a miraculous phenomenon to behold. Indeed, their electrical activities, including diastolic depolarization and automaticity (properties that confer on them their pacemaking behavior), are unparalleled in cellular physiology.

Complicating the significant attrition of pacemaker cells with age is the increased deposition of adipose tissue, amyloid, and collagen that leads to sinoatrial nodal disease. Comparable phenomena (attrition and disease) are also observed in the atrioventricular node, the bundle of His, left and right bundle branches, Purkinje fibers, and other cells of the specialized electrical conduction system of the heart. In aging, the duration of a cardiac action potential and thus the longevity of the accompanying ventricular contraction are prolonged due to the extended release of calcium ions. Mechanistically, prolongation is caused by slower inactivation of L-type calcium channels in the cell membrane, and by decreased efflux of potassium ions from inside the cell. Also, calcium reuptake by the sarcoplasmic reticulum, an intracellular organelle that plays a key role in calcium homeostasis and thus in excitation-contraction coupling, is decreased, while activity of the sodium-calcium exchanger is increased.

The Aging Blood Vessels

Blood vessels come in a variety of locations, sizes, and functions. They also have markedly different names. Consider all of the vessels to be found either in the pulmonary or systemic circulatory systems. Think of them as being arranged in beds that are both in series and in parallel to one another. Now imagine them to be located either on the arterial or venous sides of the circulation. The arterial and venous blood vessels are separated by true capillaries and other microcirculatory vessels (the microcirculation). Finally, most blood vessels are so small that they cannot be seen with the unaided eye (for example, the true capillaries), but others are so large that your little finger could be inserted in their lumina (such as the trunks of the aorta and the pulmonary artery).

This picture gives one a realistic view of the anatomical arrangement of blood vessels. However, it cannot help one understand the influences of aging on them. It is the intimate morphological details of vessel walls, the nerves that innervate them, the physiological functions of each segment of vessel, and the pliable elastic elements and rigid noncompliant elements that help define the aging process in blood vessels. Collectively, it is these things that will determine, in part, how your blood pressure, blood flow, and resistance to blood flow change with age.

As a cardiovascular physiologist, I wish everyone could measure his or her own hemodynamics over time and keep accurate records. Hemodynamics is the physics and physiology of blood pressure, blood flow, and resistance to blood flow. The first two aspects of hemodynamics, blood pressure and blood flow, can be measured directly and indirectly. The last, resistance to blood flow, cannot be measured directly or indirectly; instead, it is a calculated variable. Resistance is the quotient of blood pressure divided by blood flow. If blood pressure is measured in units of millimeters of mercury (mmHg) and blood flow in milliliters per minute (mL/min), then resistance to blood flow is calculated as pressure divided by flow and expressed in units of mmHg/mL/min.

If one is interested in comparing, for example, the resistances in a small woman and a large man, then the units of mmHg/mL/min can be normalized or corrected for kilograms (kg) of body weight. In this case the units of expression would be mmHg/mL/min/kg. In this way, we can make a valid comparison between a woman weighing 100 pounds and a man weighing 200 pounds. Similarly, if a physiologist is comparing blood flow in a large organ (weighing kilograms) with that in a small organ (weighing only grams), the comparison would be valid only if the data were normalized for tissue weight. These concepts become important as we age because many of us gain weight; some of us lose weight; and some maintain their weight.

What are the hallmarks of the aging blood vessel, and how might such changes affect our circulatory systems and well-being as we age? Tortuous arteries and veins are commonly observed in aging humans and animals. (Tortuous means sharp curves and angulations in a single blood vessel or in several vessels that are arranged in series.) Although mild tortuosity (a single gradual curve or angulation) is of little concern, severe tortuosity can lead to ischemia. Clinical observations have linked tortuous vasculature with atherosclerosis, hypertension, and diabetes in the aging. For example, tortuosity and angulation of the internal carotid artery were observed in 35 percent and 5 percent, respectively, of 1,438 consecutive patients in one study. The internal carotid artery is one of the main supplies of cerebral blood flow. Tortuosity and angulation can cause the blood flow to the brain to become turbulent. This in turn can affect the circulatory or physiological homeostasis of brain function.

Tortuous femoral (leg), iliac (hip), lingual (tongue), subclavian (neck), and vertebral (brain) arteries and their branches have also been reported. Other tortuous arterial branches include those supplying the hand and fingers, skeletal muscle, and the heart (for example, in the coronary arteries of patients with hypertension and myocardial infarction). Tortuosity has been reported in retinal and conjunctiva vessels and is common in patients with retinopathy. In addition, tortuosity occurs in veins and after bypass grafting and reconstructive vascular surgery. Tortuosity can also affect venous patency (the degree to which a vessel is open and freely allows the flow of blood through it), and, due to disease of the valves, tortuosity occurs in patients with varicose veins. Tortuosity and angulation rarely occur in children but are often reported in the elderly. Moreover, the prevalence of tortuosity in arteries is tripled in healthy people as they age and is quadrupled in aged hypertensive patients. Severely tortuous and kinked arteries hinder physiological blood flow and can lead to transient ischemic attacks.

Physiological blood flow through healthy arteries is usually streamlined and laminar. This means it flows in cylindrically arranged layers (lamina). These layers slip by one another, exchanging energy as they move. The fastest layers are found in the center of the vessel, and the slowest at or near the vessel wall. Under such conditions, flow is not turbulent. Turbulence is caused by eddies of flow occurring at angles to the central axis of flow. Turbulence can lead to clumping of red blood cells, platelets, and other plasma-borne substances. Under the worst conditions, turbulence leads to the formation of intravascular clots, a potentially life-threatening pathophysiological condition.

Recent clinical studies have demonstrated that elevated blood pressure is a risk factor for the tortuosity of arteries. Mechanistically, there is some evidence to suggest that tortuosity results from the mechanical instability and remodeling that accompany tissue injury (for example, sprained ankles, twisted or strained knee joints, and jammed thumbs). The elderly are more prone to such injuries, although they are ubiquitous especially among more active populations (for example, players of basketball, field hockey, and lacrosse).

One way to minimize the chance of untoward circulatory events happening in angulated, kinked, and tortuous blood vessels is to avoid assuming fixed positions for too long. For example, do not sit in front of your computer screen for lengthy periods. After an hour or two, get up and walk a bit. This will stretch the kinked blood vessels in your previously bent knees. When on flights lasting more than a few hours, go to the restroom, walk the aisles, or brace your hands against the overhead bins and rise periodically to your tiptoes. These activities will improve blood flow in your previously kinked legs and will reduce the chance of blood clots forming there. Be proactive about the health of your aging cardiovascular system.

In December 2013 my wife and I took a twelve-hour train ride from Charlotte, North Carolina, to Philadelphia, Pennsylvania. After a couple hours of sitting, we walked from one car to another. Between this activity and going to the bathroom, we did not sit for more than two or three hours at a time. As I walked through the train, I could not help notice a few people who never moved from their seats. For example, one young mother with three children, one a fussy one- or two-year-old, never got out of her seat. If the children needed anything brought to them, the man traveling with them went to get it. In a conversation with him, I learned that they were traveling from Charlotte to New York. After twelve hours my wife and I got off in Philadelphia. Those people still had another hour or more to sit.

Aging Collateral Blood Vessels

The most important mechanism by which our circulatory systems compensate for the reduced blood flow caused by an obstructed or chronically tortuous artery is through the collateral circulation. Collateral blood vessels are defined as vascular branches off of an adjacent arterial tree (mainstream arteries) that connect the proximal part of an artery compromised by atherosclerosis or blood clot to the downstream, segmental component lying distal to an obstruction. Thus, when the mainstream artery is obstructed or partially occluded, blood flow to the ischemic tissue is supplied by collateral blood vessels. Important as the collateral circulation is, it is often incapable of restoring flow to physiological rates at rest, and it is usually incapable of delivering the augmented flow required by exercise or increased metabolic demands. This is evident by the frequency of patients with coronary or peripheral arterial disease (PAD) who experience angina or claudication on exertion. The limited capacity to restore full flow at high metabolic demands poses quality-of-life concerns to aging individuals who have chronic arterial obstruction.

In the United States alone, 300,000–900,000 patients have persistent coronary arterial angina despite repeated attempts to manage their condition medically. Angina can be any physical manifestation of inadequate coronary blood flow (acute or chronic, such as sudden or more lasting pain in the neck, shoulder, arm, chest, or back; or a sudden general feeling of not being well; or throwing up whether or not the patient has recently ingested a meal). Studies in both humans and laboratory animals demonstrate that the clinical outcome of acute arterial obstruction is worse in subjects with a poor collateral circulation than in those with a robust one. It is also conceivable that the presence of cardiovascular risk factors, including aging, causes marked deterioration of collateral circulation, significantly impairing the capacity of the collaterals to respond to the therapy. One of the best things a person can do to increase or improve collateral blood flow is to be active. Active limbs, hearts, and brains tend to have more collateral blood flow than inactive organs do. Here is another opportunity for the reader to compare Senior Olympians (see chapter 8) with their counterparts who either choose or are forced to lead lives of physical inactivity.

In a study of a small group of patients with normal coronary arteries who were undergoing replacement of their aortic valves, researchers found that all of the subjects had retrograde flow (upstream or reverse flow), measured downstream of an obstructing intracoronary balloon. About one-third of the subjects had flow values similar to patients with documented coronary artery disease, although none of the subjects had evidence of occluding atherosclerosis or stenosis. Even though collateral blood flow was variable in the subjects, immediately after balloon-induced coronary artery occlusion, one-fifth had sufficient collateral flow to prevent myocardial ischemia. Thus, coronary collaterals are present in humans before arterial obstructive disease develops, and there is wide variation in the functional capacity of such collaterals. Moreover, there is little or no evidence of those who permanently live at high altitude (such as Peruvians in the Andes and the Sherpas in the Himalayas) dying of heart attack or myocardial infarction. The few studies available reveal that all such people have hypoxia-induced, well-developed coronary collateral circulations.

About ten years ago, researchers first reported a finding that was subsequently confirmed: aging decreases the recovery of collateral-dependent blood flow following acute obstruction of arteries. Just as there are multiple processes involved in enhancing collateral blood flow, so there are many changes during aging that impair each of these processes. Such changes interfere with the capacity of collateral vessels to fully compensate for impaired flow following occlusion of arteries. Data from research with mice, for example, indicate strong genetic determinants of the numbers and diameters of collateral blood vessels and their abilities to adjust to disease and tissue injury (that is, to remodel themselves). Investigators demonstrated that in the mouse hind limb, aging causes decreases in both the number and diameter of collateral blood vessels. These and other changes impaired the ability of the hind limb of the mouse to recover from injury. Similar changes as well as collateral tortuosity occurred in the cerebral circulation of aging mice; they had been reported earlier in aging rats and cats. Such alterations in the cerebral circulation resulted in a sixfold increase in calculated collateral vascular resistance, and they were accompanied by an increase in the severity of experimentally induced stroke. However, rarefaction of collaterals (or reduced density of vessels) was not accompanied by loss of arterioles or capillaries in the cerebral circulation of these animals.

The major mechanism initiating change in collateral function and structure subsequent to arterial occlusion is the increased flow-induced strain imposed on the inside lining of the collateral vessels. Before obstruction of an artery, native collaterals that connect adjacent arterial trees are small (their inside diameter is 20–40 micrometers) and have high resistance. No net pressure gradient exists between two adjacent sets of vessels under resting conditions. This has been shown by near-zero collateral blood flow under baseline conditions. A subsequent obstruction of a main artery reduces downstream pressure in that artery and its branches. This results in a pressure gradient with increased flow between downstream arteries and the interconnecting, collateral vessels. The increased flow and strain on the lining of the vessel wall (the endothelium) can cause release of adhesion molecules, damaging oxidants, vasoactive molecules, and pro-inflammatory genes. Such cellular and molecular events, accompanied by tissue ischemia, can result in mobilization of stem, progenitor, and inflammatory cells that contribute to remodeling of the vasculature and ischemic tissue.

Early investigations of aging-related vascular changes focused on large arteries. However, more recent investigations have measured the diameters of collateral vessels in the mouse hind limb and brain before and several days after acute occlusion of the main arteries supplying these organs. In this species, aging reduces collateral function and structure in both vascular beds. Unfortunately, there are no studies in humans that focus specifically on the effects of aging on collateral remodeling. This is due, in part, to difficulty in measuring collaterals or collateral-dependent flow in humans, and to lack of choice among patients. The few experiments that have been conducted have focused exclusively on subjects with coronary artery disease. Of course, this was before the recently developed interest in PAD in humans. Collateral blood flow in coronary patients is critically influenced by the longevity and magnitude of vessel obstruction. For example, researchers analyzed data collected on hundreds of patients with total occlusions of the coronary arteries related to infarction within seventy-two hours of their heart attacks. After statistically eliminating other contributing factors, the researchers concluded that advanced age independently predicted impaired collateral circulation.

Another important question that has clinical implications is the time period in which aging-induced deterioration in collateral function occurs. Does it occur gradually over a lifetime, or does it occur quickly, which would mean that it is physiologically important only in the later years or decades of life? For example, in people who have diabetes, PAD is thought to develop concurrently with the diabetes. If deterioration of the collateral circulation in limbs corresponds to the development of diabetes, then the deterioration must occur only in the later decades of life. An exception, of course, would be juvenile-onset diabetes, whose marked increase we are currently witnessing. In this case, it could be that collateral deterioration takes place over a short period of time in obese children and adolescents.

Genetics and Calories, Aging, and Cardiovascular Intersections

Geneticists studying cardiovascular disease at or near the University of Utah have been said to be in an enviable position. Salt Lake City and Salt Lake County currently have large populations of Mormons. The ancestors of these Mormons began arriving in that area about 1847. For the next fifty years, many Mormons practiced polygamy. In some cases, leaders of the religion had more than fifteen wives.

Today descendants of those polygamous families are still living in that area. Arguably, such descendants have grown up in the same environment but have different genes because their ancestors had the same father but different mothers, which means that environmental conditions that might have influenced aging and cardiovascular disease can be ruled out as the cause of differences that occur after several generations. That leaves genetics playing the lead role in the physiology and health, behavior, education, and socioeconomic outcomes of the descendants. It could even be argued that among such residents of northern Utah, genetics plays the major role in determining longevity and rates of cardiovascular and other diseases.

One of the main determinants of cardiovascular health is a person's age. By 2030 approximately 20 percent of the US population will be sixty-five years or older. For the baby boomers (those born in the period 1946–63), cardiovascular disease will be the cause of 40 percent of all deaths and will be the leading cause of death, and the overall cost of treating the disease will triple from about 2010 to 2030. Until recently the fields of cardiovascular disease and the molecular biology of aging have largely remained separate. Most rodent studies of atherosclerosis or diseases of the heart have been done in young mice, and they have taken place only in the past two or three decades. During those years scientists developing genetic and pharmacological interventions designed to extend the human life span rarely assessed whether or not those interventions improved the rate of cardiovascular disease. Fortunately, that separation is changing.

The percentage of people who are age sixty-five are older is growing rapidly. This should not be surprising when one considers the marked decline in birth rates and the increasing ages of women giving birth for the first time. Also within this age group, cardiovascular disease will remain the leading cause of death, and the cost associated with treatment of cardiovascular disease will continue to increase. These facts might be surprising when one realizes that the leading edge of the baby boomers were born at a time when cardiovascular disease was not even listed among the top ten causes of death in the United States, circa 1946–47. Of course at that time pathogenic infections and lack of pharmaceuticals for treating them were still prevalent. Moreover, we had just passed through two world wars and a flu pandemic that decimated large populations in short periods of time. Most of those lost were male.

Being male and aging are two of the greatest risk factors for developing cardiovascular disease. Although numerous cardiovascular investigations have considered both young and aged humans, there are still many unanswered questions. For example, how do the genetic pathways that regulate aging in organisms such as fruit flies, *C. elegans*, and mice apply to cardiovascular aging in humans? Likewise, in the molecular biology of aging, few studies have fully assessed the role of genetic pathways in cardiovascular health. This is due, in part, to the fact that modern molecular biologists are neither trained nor experienced in the field of classic cardiovascular physiology. Today, for example, we know of many genes and their corresponding proteins that are involved in both aging and cardiovascular health. Some of the key genes and proteins that help regulate cardiovascular health and longevity are adenosine monophosphate–activated protein kinase, insulin-like growth factor I, mammalian target of rapamycin, and the sirtuin family of molecules. Many more genes and proteins will be discovered as collaborative work in these two disciplines intensifies.

In both the aging and cardiovascular fields, it is generally accepted that diets low in calories, combined with generous physical activity, increase one's overall health and longevity. Obesity—that is, a body mass index equal to or greater than twenty-five—and a sedentary lifestyle have the opposite effects. The traditional view is that cardiovascular disease and ill health result, in part, from the accumulation of cholesterol and fatty acids and the minerals and electrolytes that they trap in tissues, particularly in the walls of blood vessels. This compromises vascular and tissue function and stimulates the production of inflammatory molecules and damaging oxidants. Diets high in calories and lifestyles with little or no physical activity might be harmful because, alone or in combination, they suppress the expression of longevity genes that promote cellular defenses against aging and disease.

The relatively new concept expressed above has its beginnings in an observation made about 1935: reducing a rat's intake of calories by 20–40 percent markedly extended its longevity. Since then, the ability of reduced calories to extend longevity has been observed in dogs, fish, monkeys, rodents, and yeast. There are exceptions, however, including various inbred and outbred strains of mice as well as field and house mice. In mammals, restricting the daily intake of calories reduces the incidence of most age-related diseases, including cancer, kidney failure, muscle wasting, and weakness. Whether or not reduced calories increase the life span of humans and subhuman primates (with the exception of macaque monkeys) is still debated, in part because of conflicting data.

The Japanese in Okinawa consume 1,785 calories per day on average. This is only a modest reduction from the US Department of Agriculture's recommendation of 2,000 calories per day for Americans, but Okinawans have lower rates of coronary heart disease and a relatively high frequency of centenarians, compared to Americans. Consistent with these data on humans, other experimental subjects who have consumed a reduced number of calories for six months to eight years reveal evidence of improved cardiovascular physiology and health, including lower blood pressure, reduced inflammatory markers, decreased oxidative stress, and reduced triglycerides.

At the beginning of January 2013, I weighed 182 pounds. This was an increase from the 175 pounds I had been maintaining for many years. My blood pressure was about 135/85 mmHg, and my blood glucose was 95 mg/dL. I was upset with my excess consumption of food (and the wrong kinds of calories) during the preceding Thanksgiving and Christmas holidays. I resolved to quickly shed the weight and dropped to 170 pounds in the next eight weeks. I did this by being careful and by trying to consume fewer calories at each meal and during each day. During that time I also weighed myself every morning at the same time and on the same scales. Each loss of half a pound or so reinforced my determination to keep going.

During that exercise in loss of weight, and while teaching laboratory students about blood glucose and the cardiovascular system in March and April 2013, I had them routinely measure their own and my blood pressure and blood glucose. After I lost those excess pounds, my blood pressure dropped to 125/80 mmHg and my blood glucose was about 80 mg/dL. I not only felt better, but as a cardiovascular physiologist I also knew how much better off my heart, blood vessels, kidneys, liver, and other organs and tissues were because of the changes. Also, I did not have to consider myself borderline hypertensive once my blood pressure returned to more favorable physiological values. I have maintained the lower weight, and I encourage most readers to shed ten or fifteen pounds in the next few months (or faster if able) and then consider whether or not it has improved their outlook on life.

Many of the fundamental molecular processes involved in protecting one's cardiovascular system by reducing food consumption are known. Restricting the intake of calories increases mitochondrial function while reducing oxidative stress in the vasculature and elsewhere. It does this, in part, by inducing the expression of specific stress response factors. The stress response factors in turn amplify the expression of the mitochondrial enzymes that are needed to maintain the physiological homeostasis of this important subcellular organelle. Reducing the intake of calories in both rodents and humans also minimizes inflammation, by suppressing the expression of vascular adhesion molecules and inflammatory cytokines such as the prostanoids. Health of the vascular endothelium is likewise enhanced by reducing one's intake of calories, and atherosclerosis and hardening of the arteries are reduced in both rodents and humans. Restricting calories also delays the onset of age-related decline in ventricular diastolic filling. This corresponds to reduced edema and inflammation and to decreased rates of ventricular diseases such as cardiomyopathy, cardiac fibrosis, and myocardial degeneration.

Aging and Blood Electrolytes

The physiological balance of electrolytes is essential to the healthy function of nerves and muscles and the heart and blood vessels. Physiolocially, the most important electrolytes are: calcium (Ca^{2+}), bicarbonate (HCO_3^-), chloride (Cl^-), hydrogen (H^+), potassium (K^+), and sodium (Na^+). There are others, but space precludes an inclusive list here. In the body, electrolytes exist in both ionized and nonionized states. The ionized state means they carry either positive or negative charges. Nonionized electrolytes do not carry charges because they are bound to other chemicals, and their electrical charges are neutralized. The numbers of charged electrolytes inside and outside of cells must be balanced. Among other disturbances, abnormalities can generate cardiac arrhythmias even if the cardiac structure and function are normal otherwise. Many of the prescription medications that the elderly take have known side effects, including potential disturbances in the balance of electrolytes.

Hypokalemia (reduced circulating concentrations of potassium ions) is the most common electrolyte abnormality found in clinical practice in the elderly. Physiological concentrations of potassium outside the cells (including in the blood) are about 4.5 milliequivalents per liter (mEq/L). Potassium values less than 3.6 mEq/L are seen in over 20 percent of hospitalized patients. Up to 40 percent of patients on diuretics and almost 50 percent of patients resuscitated from ventricular fibrillation have low potassium levels. Hypokalemia usually results from decreased potassium intake, including the reduced food consumption that is often seen in the elderly either because they refuse to eat, forget to eat, or can't feed themselves. Hypokalemia also results from increased excretion by the kidneys. The electrophysiological effects of hypokalemia predispose the heart to arrhythmias that can be life threatening.

Although less common than hypokalemia, hyperkalemia (concentrations of potassium in the blood that are greater than 4.5 mEq/L) might be even more serious and can also affect the elderly, among other groups. Hyperkalemia affects approximately 8 percent of hospitalized patients in the United States. It is most commonly associated with failure of the kidneys. When potassium concentrations reach levels of 5.5–7.0 mEq/L, multiple disturbances in the electrocardiogram can be seen. These include tall-peaked, narrow-based T waves (an electrocardiogram sign of disturbed cardiac electrophysiology). At levels of 10 mEq/L or greater, marked intraventricular conduction delay, ventricular tachycardia, ventricular fibrillation, and even cardiac arrest can occur. Hyperkalemia results from either decreased excretion by the kidneys or a transfer of potassium from inside to outside the cell (malfunctioning cell membranes).

Hypocalcemia (reduced extracellular calcium) is most frequently seen in the setting of chronic renal insufficiency and is usually associated with other electrolyte abnormalities. As a consequence of low intracellular calcium, the contractility of skeletal, cardiac, vascular, and visceral smooth muscle decreases. Moreover, hypocalcemia can affect cardiac cells differently and can increase excitability of the cells by a direct action on their membranes. Sustained lack of calcium in the elderly or any malnourished person can hasten muscle wasting. In contrast, elevated extracellular calcium has a stabilizing effect on the cell membrane, can strengthen the force of muscle contraction, and can increase heart rate modestly.

Sodium is the most abundant positively charged electrolyte outside the cell, and it determines how rapidly a cell responds once it is electrically activated. Sodium's movement into the cell increases precipitously with the initiation of an action potential. Elevated extracellular sodium increases, and reduced sodium decreases, the cell's electrical response. High sodium levels prolong the duration of action potentials. Despite the frequency of sodium abnormalities, particularly inadequate salt intake in the elderly, its electrophysiological effects are rarely of clinical significance.

Imbalances in electrolytes in the elderly can have life-threatening consequences, including cardiac arrest and sudden cardiac death (hyperkalemia). Of course, the weaker one's heart is, the lower the concentration of excess potassium needed to do serious damage. The diets and daily nutrition of the elderly must be carefully monitored. A simple change in the content of body water can lead to an imbalance in electrolytes and potentially grave consequences. Seniors must be helped to ensure that they have an adequate water intake from all sources (direct, indirect, and intrinsic water).

10

The Aging Respiratory System

My wife and I were sitting in the ophthalmologist's office waiting for my appointment. We struck up a conversation with another couple who were in their early eighties. While her husband was being examined, the woman told us of a recent experience and then warned us not to turn seventy ("it's all downhill from age seventy").

It seems that this woman had returned home after doing errands and was unhappy with the way she had parked in the driveway. She started the car, intending to back up and then park in a better position. Instead of shifting into reverse, she unwittingly shifted into drive. As the car began moving she could tell that it was going in the wrong direction. She knew she had to apply the brake but instead applied the accelerator. Confused and anxious, she tried to apply more force to the brake pedal, but instead applied it to the accelerator. She drove into the front of the house and adjoining garage, doing considerable damage but luckily injuring no one (her husband was inside but out of harm's way).

As a result, this woman had to surrender her driver's license. She and her husband complained about her loss of independence and his newly acquired responsibilities. During our conversation, the woman told us that she had been diagnosed with sleep apnea and reported that, during sleeping hours, her frequency of apnea (cessation of breathing) happened every few minutes.

greater in the expiratory intercostal muscles than in the inspiratory ones. This means that expiration, which is passive except during exertion, is likely to become impaired with aging before inspiration does.

There seems to be no age-related change in the thickness of the diaphragm, even though structural changes in the chest wall reduce the curvature and maximal pressure gradient that exists across the diaphragm. In addition, the width of the esophageal hiatus (the junction where the esophagus passes through the diaphragm into the abdomen) is greater after the age of seventy years. This suggests that the elderly are more likely to develop conditions such as hiatal hernia. That possibility is one reason why older people who have persistent pain in the chest cavity and upper abdomen should seek medical advice.

Moreover, maximal static inspiratory and expiratory pressures decrease with age, reflecting a reduction in the strength of all respiratory muscles. Also, the time lag between the stimulation of the phrenic nerve and the contraction of the diaphragm (latency) increases with age, whereas the amplitudes of action potentials in the phrenic nerve decrease. The latter changes might represent degeneration of insulation of nerve fibers, which could lead to reduced contractile strength of the diaphragm. In addition, atrophy and loss of fast-twitch muscle fibers in the diaphragm of the elderly occur with age.

The results of experiments on laboratory animals can be informative. Analysis of isolated phrenic nerve-diaphragm preparations from aged rats has identified changes in respiratory physiology that we have not been able to confirm in elderly humans. Phrenic nerve axons innervating fast-twitch muscle fibers that are recruited later in the contractile process during inspiration are smaller in older rats than in younger ones, but surface areas at the nerve terminals are greater. Smaller nerve fibers conduct action potentials at slower rates and could therefore delay the contraction of respiratory muscles. However, this could be compensated for by the larger neuromuscular junctions, which conceivably would release more neurotransmitters and therefore activate more muscles. Together, these changes could represent an attempt to maintain maximal force of inspiratory contraction during aging.

What happens to the size of respiratory neurons in the phrenic nerve of humans with age is unknown and will remain so pending developments in technology and experimentation. In humans, the density of connections between intercostal muscles and corresponding respiratory motor nerves increases with age. So do branching and enlargement of the postjunctional areas of contact between nerves and muscles. Similar to changes occurring at the neuromuscular junction of the aging rat diaphragm, the structural alterations in humans mostly reflect junctional degeneration and compromised contractile function.

In addition to the age-related atrophy of intercostal muscles and the deterioration of neuromuscular junctions, calcification of cartilage in the rib cage and vertebral columns—coupled with osteoporosis—contributes to reduced compliance of the chest wall as we get older. After about age fifty, elastin fibers in the bronchioles are disrupted and lost, and the structural integrity of collagen and elastin is reduced. Alveoli become wider and shallower, with flattened inner surfaces; alveolar ducts are dilated. After about age thirty-five, there is a gradual increase in the stiffness of the pulmonary vasculature. In association with this structural remodeling of the vascular wall, pulmonary arterial and pulmonary wedge pressures become significantly elevated after age fifty. In addition, the capability of the lungs for gas exchange is compromised, as the volume and numbers of pulmonary capillaries decrease. However, the content of the surfactant and its physiological properties do not appear to be affected by age. This suggests that type II alveolar cells, although fewer in number and much larger than type I alveolar cells, remain physiologically intact during the aging process.

The nasopharynx shows significant physical changes as resistance to airflow through the nasal passages increases with age. There is an age-related decrease in cartilage-producing cells, but there are no known alterations in the integrity of the mucosal lining (nasal secretions), functions of the nasal turbinates, or the structure and function of the nasal cilia. Differences in pharyngeal size and tone do exist between young and older adults. The posterior pharyngeal wall is thinner and does not contract to the same extent in older adults as in young ones. Pharyngeal relaxation is phasic during inspiration and is greater in older than in younger men during waking hours. With age-related reductions in muscle mass, the pharyngeal airway is more collapsible in older people, leading to increased airway resistance.

Airway structural volume, particularly in men, increases with age in association with increased soft tissue, while upper airway volume decreases.

Structural changes in laryngeal muscle are observable beginning at about sixty years of age. For example, in the thyroarytenoid musculature (which helps operate the voice box, and therefore affects the volume, tone, and endurance of the voice) there is a marked increase in connective tissue along with pathologic changes in muscle fibers, including evidence of mutation of mitochondrial DNA. Hardening of the laryngeal skeleton is also evident with increasing age. These—and corresponding changes in nerves such as the recurrent laryngeal nerves, which operate the musculature of the vocal cords—can result in incomplete closure of the glottis secondary to bowing of the vocal folds. This has the potential for compromising respiratory and protective functions of the larynx, as well as weakening the voice. If you are a teacher, singer, or other frequent user of the voice, take care early in your career to protect this vital function for later years (for example, don't strain your voice, use microphones or speakers where and when possible; and use fewer words and shorter sentences in your verbal conversations). In my late fifties or early sixties, I was diagnosed with right-sided vocal cord paresis (partial paralysis). Since then, my voice has never been as strong as it once was, or had its former endurance. I have been teaching for more than forty years, which of course requires me to use my voice a great deal.

Ventilation, Perfusion, and the Consumption of Oxygen

Another strength in the marvelous design of our mysterious bodies is the matching of blood flow with air flow. In healthy young adults, the volume of blood passing through the lungs each minute (about 4–6 liters) is equal to the volume of air passing through the air sacs during the same period of time. We call this equality of blood and air flow the ventilation-to-perfusion ratio and abbreviate it V_A/Q. V_A stands for alveolar ventilation and Q represents cardiac output, or total blood flow. A ventilation-to-perfusion ratio of about one means that all regions of both lungs are adequately ventilated with air and perfused with blood.

A change in the ratio can mean one of several things: the supply of air can be too little or too much, the supply of blood can be too great or too small, or both air and blood can be present in the wrong quantities. Any mismatching of ventilation and perfusion in the lungs can ultimately affect all body tissues, including the brain, heart, and other vital organs. Moreover, the ratio is modestly affected by body position—that is, when we stand upright, ventilation and perfusion values are a bit different from those when we are lying down. This is because of the height of the lungs, the mass of air and blood, and the influence of gravity. The overall effect can mean less efficient matching of lung ventilation and perfusion in the apex and base of the lungs in one position than in another.

In addition to the potential mismatching of air and blood flow, the partial pressure of oxygen in arterial blood (arterial PO_2) decreases progressively with age. This is important because it is the dissolved oxygen in the blood and other fluids of the body that creates a partial pressure and drives the movement of oxygen from one site to the next (for example, across the walls of systemic capillaries and into the cells). However, with aging, alveolar PO_2 in well-ventilated regions of the lungs does not change, and therefore the alveolar–arterial oxygen difference [$(A–a)dO_2$] increases progressively. Alveolar dead space (regions of the lung and pulmonary circulation where gas exchange does not take place) increases in association with reduced pulmonary blood flow. Alveolar dead space and the ventilation-perfusion mismatch that takes place in or near it both increase with age. This is because there is a greater tendency for closure of the airways in the lower lung regions, where there is less elastic tissue in older humans to hold them open. This can lead to a substantial percentage of airways being closed, thereby producing a low V_A/Q ratio during normal breathing.

Compounding the problem of ventilation-perfusion mismatching is the decreasing volume of gas that diffuses across the membranes between the alveoli and pulmonary capillaries with age (pulmonary diffusion capacity). Loss of alveolar surface area and decreased blood volume in pulmonary capillaries are responsible for this decline. Thus, the partial pressure of oxygen in systemic arterial blood decreases progressively from about 95 mmHg at age twenty to about 75 mmHg at age seventy, a significant difference between young and old people.

Although the partial pressure of oxygen in systemic arterial blood declines with age, the partial pressure of carbon dioxide in the same blood is maintained. It has been hypothesized that decreasing resting and basal metabolic rates and an increasing diffusion capacity of carbon dioxide across the alveolar-capillary barrier explain this. However, another likely explanation is the mismatching of ventilation and perfusion in different regions of the lungs with age. Also, neurogenic control of ventilation is more sensitive to elevations in the partial pressure of arterial carbon dioxide than to reductions in the partial pressure of arterial oxygen.

Even without impediments such as chronic obstructive pulmonary disease (also called chronic bronchitis and emphysema), small airways collapse more easily as we age. Collectively, these age-related degenerative changes lead to atelectasis (collapse of the alveoli), inadequate ventilation, and declining oxygenation of the blood. This is evidenced by the decrease in partial pressure of oxygen in arterial blood under resting, baseline conditions in the elderly. Reduced partial pressure of oxygen is important because the difference in partial pressures of oxygen in the atmosphere, the lung, and the blood ultimately drives the delivery of oxygen to the tissues and cells. As partial pressure gradients decrease, so does the delivery of oxygen.

There are many ways to estimate lung function, and these can be used in both young healthy adults and in aging unhealthy people. One of the most important tests is called maximum oxygen consumption (VO_{2max}). This is the maximal amount of oxygen that a person can consume in one minute. It is influenced by several variables, not the least important of which is the strength of the muscles used in respiration. The physical condition of the diaphragm; the muscles between the ribs; and the auxiliary muscles of respiration, including those in the abdomen, back, neck, and shoulders help determine how much oxygen we can take in. Of course, as I have already pointed out, muscles atrophy and lose mass, tone, and strength as we age.

There are different ways to estimate maximum oxygen consumption. The gold standard is using treadmills and physiological equipment such as oxygen electrodes. I will describe a typical test, like the ones I have experienced. The subject arrives at a university's human performance laboratory or a hospital's respiratory unit, often early in the morning. He (or she) is well hydrated and has been fasting for twelve to eighteen hours. He changes into exercise attire, is asked to rest for a brief period (perhaps fifteen to thirty minutes), and is instrumented. This process can include inserting a catheter into an easily accessible arm vein to collect blood samples. It also includes wearing fitted headgear that supports a face mask connected to both oxygen and carbon dioxide monitors. Baseline data are collected as he stands motionless on the treadmill. These data include heart rate, respiratory rate, volume of airflow during each respiratory cycle, inhaled partial pressure of oxygen (in the room air), and exhaled partial pressure of carbon dioxide. A nurse or technician collects a sample of venous blood during this period.

Once baseline data are collected, the investigator turns the treadmill on, and the belt begins moving at a slow, predetermined velocity. The subject walks at a slow pace while the investigator monitors the above variables. After two or three minutes, the speed of the treadmill is increased, and the subject is forced to walk at a faster pace. After two or three such increments, the subject is forced to jog to keep pace with the moving belt. Then the slope of the treadmill, which was parallel with the surface of the floor, is changed incrementally. Soon the subject is forced to run uphill until he is exhausted. At this point, he grasps the rails of the treadmill, lifts his body off the moving belt, and supports himself momentarily while the slope and speed of the machine are returned to baseline. During the entire period, including the state of exhaustion, the nurse or technician collects data. After the treadmill is stopped, the subject is carefully escorted to a chair, where he is seated while the nurse or technician collects postexercise samples of blood. The test is then completed, and the subject is allowed to recover for twenty or thirty minutes.

While I was writing the first draft of this chapter, I was making improvements to the experiments that my colleagues and I conduct in Systems Physiology Laboratory at Rutgers University. A co-worker and her husband had just returned from a vacation in Alberta, Canada. They had visited Lake Louise and Banff, hiked in several provincial parks, and taken a whitewater rafting trip. Both of them are about my age and are in good physical condition, but they are acclimated to the sea-level conditions of central New Jersey. My co-worker commented about their diminished strength and endurance as they hiked and engaged in other physical activities in Alberta. I remarked that one cause might have been the climate and altitude, but that another could have been their ages. Neither of them had engaged in these physical activities in the Canadian Rockies before, and their judgments of endurance were probably based on hikes in New Jersey, where elevations do not exceed approximately 1,800 feet. In addition, the climate of the Canadian Rockies is less humid than that of the East Coast.

While exerting themselves in the Canadian Rockies, my co-worker and her husband could have experienced marginal, high-altitude pulmonary conditions that would have affected their abilities to perform, including high altitude pulmonary edema, high altitude cerebral edema, and generalized mountain sickness without the edema and/or ischemia. Each of these conditions involves reduced oxygenation and is more prevalent in the unconditioned elderly than in the conditioned and younger person.

On another occasion, my wife and children and I were visiting Mount Timpanogos Cave in the Wasatch Range of the Rocky Mountains, just east of Provo, Utah. We were with a tour group and had just completed a vertical climb of 1,100 feet and were resting and waiting to enter the cave. It was about 11:30 A.M., and I was in my late forties. The children were restless and getting hungry, and my wife reminded me that we had left our packed lunches in the car. She asked me to quickly go back down and return with them before the tour entered the cave, about noon. The trail was paved and consisted of a lengthy series of switchbacks, or periodic changes of direction, each amounting to about 180 degrees and extending the 1,100 vertical feet to a linear distance of about a mile and a half. I jogged down, retrieved the lunches, and began slowly jogging back up.

The base of the trail is about 6,700 feet above sea level; the mouth of the cave, therefore, is at 7,800 feet. After jogging perhaps a quarter of the way up, I became exhausted and stopped to rest, lowering my head to my knees. When I raised my head, I was confused and disoriented. I could not tell which sections of the trail ascended and which descended. I was nervous and wondered if I could return to my family in time. About this time some passersby appeared, and I asked them to orient me. They pointed to the cave, and I thanked them but sat still for several more minutes. I should have been surprised that no one offered assistance, but I wasn't. After a few more minutes I was able to slowly and carefully make my way back to the cave and to my family. My wife was surprised that I had taken so long. I was relieved to have escaped further vertigo and the marginal effects of acute mountain sickness.

For more in-depth reading on this topic (expeditions and mountain sickness in climbers young and old), I direct the interested reader to John B. West. As a young man, West was with Sir Edmund Hillary when the summit of Everest was reached for the first time, in May 1953. Later, West organized the first research expedition to Everest to study the influence of altitude and climate on respiration and circulation in humans. West is an experimental respiratory and circulatory physiologist. His numerous research articles and multiple monographs and books on the outcome of his mountain climbing adventures are worth reading.

Tests of Lung Performance, Respiratory Mechanics, and Ventilation

The respiratory cycle arguably consists of three phases: an inspiratory phase (breathing air in), an expiratory phase (exhaling used air to the atmosphere), and an inter-respiratory interval. The last phase is the period immediately after expiration but just before inspiration, when air is flowing in neither direction.

Imagine that under resting conditions and when in good health, you respire eighteen times each minute. This means that each respiratory cycle lasts 3.3 seconds or 3,300 milliseconds. If we assume that the three phases I listed are of equal duration under physiological conditions, you would be drawing air in for about 1,100 milliseconds, exhaling air for 1,100 milliseconds, and handling no movement of air for another 1,100 milliseconds. All respiratory physiologists might not agree that there are three, rather than only two, phases in a respiratory cycle. However, if there are three phases, and since we know what is happening during the inspiratory and expiratory phases, we must ask what is going on during the inter-respiratory interval, and how are these events affected by age?

In general, respiratory performance begins to decline after age thirty. Most of the changes result from decreases in compliance of the thorax, static elastic recoil of the lungs, and strength of the respiratory muscles. This makes sense, since it is well known that elastic material in our tissues is replaced by stiffer collagen tissue as we age. Likewise, we lose muscle mass in the arms, legs, and elsewhere, so why not also in the respiratory muscles of the chest wall? There are many tests for assessing these and other functions of the lungs. The tests include measurements of both static and dynamic lung function. Lungs are static when there is no air flow—for example, at the ends of inspiration and expiration. They are dynamic when air is moving in or out. Whether dynamic or static, most measures of lung function show decreases with age.

To test static lung function, pulmonologists measure tidal volume, inspiratory reserve volume, and expiratory reserve volume, among other things. Tidal volume is the amount of air drawn in and then breathed out with each respiratory cycle. Tidal volume takes its name from the periodicity of ocean tides: the tide comes in and then goes out on a rhythmic, cyclic basis; and each wave that washes ashore follows the same path that the previous wave did. Only the volumes of water and surf change with high and low tides. Our breathing is similar: each volume inspired (and expired) follows the same path the previous volume did. Only the volumes inspired and expired are subject to change.

For a 70-kilogram person, tidal volume is about 500 milliliters under resting conditions. An unhealthy young person or an aged one will inspire less than this. Tidal volumes are quantifiable. The instrumentation and methods used are collectively referred to as spirometry. Using spirometry and continuing to test lung function, the pulmonologist estimates inspiratory and expiratory reserve volumes. To determine one's inspiratory reserve volume, the pulmonologist asks one to make a forceful inspiratory effort at the end of a normal inspiration. This is to draw in as much additional air as possible (above the 500 milliliters of tidal volume). One's expiratory reserve volume at the end of a resting expiratory effort is determined similarly (that is, one is asked to exhale as much additional air as possible). From these and appropriate data bases, the examiner can draw conclusions about the function of the patient's lungs.

Total lung capacity, or the volume of air in the lungs after a maximal inspiratory effort, is determined by the strength of the inspiratory muscles and the elastic recoil of the chest wall and lungs. Total lung capacity does not necessarily change significantly with age. This is because the decreased outward elastic recoil of the chest wall that accompanies loss of strength of respiratory muscles is compensated for by the decreased inward recoil of the lungs associated with the deterioration of elasticity of connective tissue in the airways. In other words, these two forces that oppose each other tend to decrease equally with age.

Another measure of lung function is residual volume. This is the volume of air remaining in the lungs after one expires forcefully and maximally. Residual volume increases with age as does the ratio of residual volume to total lung capacity. Residual volume also represents air that is not available for exchange with the blood. It is determined by the strength of the expiratory muscles that oppose the recoil of the chest wall at low thoracic volumes, and by the collapse of small airways and trapping of gas in the alveoli during forced expiration. With loss of strength of expiratory muscles, there is less force to oppose the recoil of the chest wall and thus an increase in residual volume.

Vital capacity is the volume of air exhaled during a maximal expiration that immediately follows a maximal inspiration. It is equal to the difference between total lung capacity and residual volume. Vital capacity decreases with age because residual volume increases while total lung capacity is unchanged. Functional residual capacity increases with age by 1 to 3 percent per decade. At functional residual capacity, the elastic forces of the lung and chest wall are equal and oriented in opposite directions.

The tissue surfaces that line the interior of the chest wall (the parietal pleura) and the exterior of the lungs (the visceral pleura, or the pleural membranes) link these two opposing forces (elastic recoil of the chest wall and lungs) across the intrapleural space. With age, the alveoli enlarge and combine, which results in losses of elasticity and surface area and an increase in the fixed lung volume. Coupled with less efficient mixing of respiratory gases and their exchange across the alveolar-capillary barrier, static relationships between pressure and volume are shifted toward reduced elastic recoil of the lungs with age. The rate of decrease in recoil of the lungs exceeds that of the chest wall so that lung volume at the end of a normal expiration increases.

Expiratory reserve volume is approximately equal to functional residual capacity. Expiratory reserve volume decreases in aging because transmural pressure (the pressure gradient across the alveolar wall) increases and causes compression of airways. The increase in transmural pressure impairs expiratory airflow and prevents the alveoli from emptying as completely as they did at younger ages. Although both functional residual capacity and residual volume increase with age, residual volume increases more.

Dynamic lung function is assessed during the actual movement of air. Imagine that a subject's filled lungs hold a maximum volume of six liters. Now imagine that he is asked to exhale as much of the six liters as possible and to do it as rapidly as possible. The pulmonologist can quantify the volume of air removed and how long it takes the subject to remove that volume. The volume removed is called the forced expiratory volume. The pulmonologist estimates the fraction of the total volume removed in the first second. This is called the forced expiratory volume in one second (FEV1). Most healthy adults can remove about 80 percent of the volume in one second. For people with unhealthy lungs (such as smokers and those with chronic bronchitis or emphysema), the volume removed is appreciably less, as it is in the aging person.

Another test of dynamic lung function evaluates maximal voluntary ventilation (MVV). This is done by asking the subject to breathe as deeply and as rapidly as possible for a brief period of time (for example, 8–12 respiratory cycles in thirty seconds). This is a challenging test because it takes concentration and considerable effort. Because of the excess volume of carbon dioxide exhaled, it can also cause dizziness and vertigo, even in a recumbent person. Both the examiner and the subject have to be cautious. During the test, the subject is also instructed to make respiratory cycles as uniform as possible. From the data collected (number of cycles, duration of the effort, tidal volume during each cycle) the pulmonologist calculates how many liters of air were moved into and out of the lungs in one minute. She can then compare the subject's results with standardized data for people of the same gender, age, size, and conditions of health. In healthy young adults, MVV can vary from as few as 50 liters (in a small woman) to more than 150 liters (in a large man). MVV declines with age.

Other measurements of the dynamic function of lungs also decrease with age, including forced vital capacity (FVC), a measure of maximal expiratory volume, and forced expiratory volume in one second (FEV1). Both FVC and FEV1 are linked to reduced compliance of the chest wall and to reduced strength of the expiratory muscles. Changes are also caused by a greater tendency of the small airways to close during forced efforts to expel air. Also, the lung volume at which the small airways begin to close during forced expiration increases. This is due, in part, to loss of the mass of respiratory muscles. As mentioned above, the intercostals and auxiliary muscles of respiration all lose mass and strength with age.

The age-related changes just described begin with decreased numbers, size, and function of respiratory neurons. For example, as reviewed in chapter 2, most aspects of nerve function decline with age. The phrenic and intercostal nerves all lose mass and function with age. Also, there is ample evidence that type II muscle fibers (such as intercostal muscles) atrophy and become fewer in number with age. Type II muscle cells are either resistant to fatigue (type IIa) or are fatigable (type IIb). As type IIa fibers become smaller and fewer, it becomes progressively more difficult for humans and other animals to successfully engage in activities that challenge the respiratory system. This is evidenced, for example, by a decline in FEV1, maximal uptake of oxygen, and partial pressure of oxygen in arterial blood in the aged. It is true of conditioned, elite competitors, even if they engage in the same competitive activities throughout a lifetime. It is much more applicable to the physically unfit.

It is noteworthy that in a comparison of older subjects (60–101 years) and younger ones (35–55 years), a linear correlation has been observed between age and latency of response in the phrenic nerve. Latency is the time that elapses between the application of a stimulus to a nerve and its response to the stimulus. Investigators have observed a prolongation of latency of 0.06 milliseconds per year of age. The increasing latency, they hypothesize, is most likely related to the degeneration of nerve axons and to the disproportionate loss of large myelinated nerve fibers. Myelin, or the nerves' insulating material, helps nerves respond more quickly to stimuli and conduct their electrical signals more rapidly. As mentioned above, the aging of peripheral nerves causes a loss in muscle strength, a change that occurs from the sixth decade onward. These results suggest that special attention should be paid to subjects over the age of sixty when they undergo investigation for disorders related to loss of insulating myelin in peripheral nerves.

Nonrespiratory Lung Functions and Age

In addition to respiration, the lungs have nonrespiratory functions. One such function is mechanical and structural. The rib cage, sternum, and vertebral column form a protective cage for the heart, great vessels, and other tissues. In the case of sudden jolts to the body and their potential damaging effects on the heart, the thorax and air-filled lungs provide protection that is analogous to that given by airbags to a person inside a car. During an automobile accident, the deployed airbags help soften the blow and reduce potential injury to the body. Inflated lungs act like deployed airbags for the delicate heart, great vessels, and other soft tissue. Aside from this obvious structural function of the thorax and air-filled lungs, there are more frequent metabolic and regulatory functions as well.

Metabolically, the walls of pulmonary capillaries produce an important enzyme called angiotensin-converting enzyme, or ACE. This enzyme is involved in the regulation of blood pressure. If systemic blood pressure decreases (including in the renal arteries), the kidneys release another enzyme called renin. In the systemic circulation, renin causes the enzymatic production of angiotensin I (AI). AI is physiologically inert. However, as AI passes through the lungs (and selected other tissues) it comes in contact with ACE and is converted to angiotensin II (AII). AII is a potent vasoconstrictor that acts on the renal and other arteries of the systemic circulation to elevate blood pressure. Collectively, this is called the renin-angiotensin system (RAS). The rise in renal blood pressure restores normal kidney function, renin is no longer released, and a new physiological steady state for systemic blood pressure is reached. Pharmaceutical companies around the world have taken advantage of this physiological knowledge by manufacturing products that inhibit ACE and therefore help control blood pressure in the aged and others.

Blood pressure is typically lower in premenopausal women than in men of the same age. However, as women go through menopause, the prevalence of hypertension increases and can even outpace that of aging men. There is mounting evidence that blood pressure might not be as well controlled in medicated women as in medicated men. Globally, 25 percent of adult women are hypertensive. In the United States, more than 75 percent of women older than sixty years of age are hypertensive, and 41 percent of younger postmenopausal women are. One mechanism by which blood pressure might rise in aging postmenopausal women is through activation of the renin-angiotensin system. When compared with premenopausal women, postmenopausal women have increased renin in their plasma as well as increased AI, AII, and ACE activity. There is also thought to be a genetic component to the RAS that contributes to postmenopausal hypertension. For example, certain abnormalities in the gene that produces renin are associated with hypertension in women ages forty to seventy years, but not in men of the corresponding ages.

Blockers of AII receptors are well tolerated, have beneficial cardiovascular and metabolic effects, and are commonly used for the treatment of
hypertension, diabetes, and stroke (all are risk factors for brain disorders).
Cell cultures show that AII blockers have direct neuroprotective effects,
and studies in animals reveal that they reduce brain ischemia, anxiety,
brain inflammation, depression, and stress-related disorders. Angiotensin
receptor blockers have also been shown, in rodents, to increase longevity.
The anti-stress, anti-ischemic, and anti-inflammatory effects of AII receptor blockers suggest that they have great therapeutic potential for a wide
range of disorders, including those associated with aging. Since inflammation of the brain is known to compound ischemia, stroke, age-associated
declines in cognition, and depression, angiotensin receptor blockers could
be used to treat neurodegenerative and traumatic disorders of the brain.
Recent clinical studies suggest that they also protect cognition after stroke
and in aging.

Women are typically more likely than men to see their health care
providers and to take their medications. Nevertheless, as noted above,
hypertension in medicated women is less well controlled than in age-
matched medicated men, suggesting that different pathophysiologic
mechanisms—perhaps even multiple concurrent mechanisms—contribute
to hypertension in postmenopausal women. Moreover, obesity, anxiety,
and depression are all higher in women at any age, than in men of corresponding ages. Obesity elevates circulating concentrations of leptin, and
obesity, leptin, aging, and anxiety all stimulate the sympathetic nervous
system. Collectively and individually, these changes place women at higher
risk of cardiovascular diseases, including hypertension. This might require
therapeutic approaches in women that are distinct from those that have
proven successful in men.

The Physiological Control of Breathing

Groups of rhythmically active neurons in respiratory regions of the brainstem control motor output to the diaphragm, intercostal muscles, upper
airways, and accessory muscles of respiration. We call these aggregates of
respiratory-related neurons "control centers." The respiratory control centers maintain a rhythmic pattern of breathing that leads to the effective

exchange of respiratory gases between lungs and the atmosphere under normal resting conditions. Interactions of the respiratory control centers with the cerebral cortex, nearby cardiovascular control centers, and visceral autonomic and skeletal muscle nerve networks allow respiratory activity to adjust to changes in posture; transitions between sleep and wakefulness; and activities such as exercise, phonation (the audible use of the voice), swallowing, coughing, and defecating.

Two sources of sensory input continuously reach the respiratory control centers to help maintain arterial partial pressures of carbon dioxide (PCO_2) and oxygen (PO_2) and pH within physiological ranges of 40–45 millimeters of mercury (mmHg), 80–100 mmHg, and 7.38–7.42, respectively. One source of input is supplied by the central chemoreceptors of the brainstem and is most active when the person is awake. The other source comes from the peripheral chemoreceptors of the carotid and aortic bodies. These chemically sensitive nerves are stimulated by changes in PO_2, PCO_2, and pH. In addition to central and peripheral chemoreceptors, chemosensitive cells have been identified in neural tissue between the brainstem and cerebral hemispheres. Of these, orexin neurons in the region of the lateral hypothalamus seem to be most strongly linked to breathing.

According to some reports, neurons of the central chemoreceptors provide 60–80 percent of the ventilatory response to changes in PCO_2 and pH, while the remainder is attributed to the peripheral chemoreceptors (that is, mainly in the carotid bodies as opposed to the aortic bodies). However, the relative contributions of central and peripheral chemoreceptors remain a matter of debate. There is evidence that at lower levels of hypercapnia (excess PCO_2, or $\geqslant$45–50 mmHg) peripheral chemoreceptors in the carotid body have a greater influence, while central chemoreceptors are more dominant at higher levels (such as 50–60 mmHg). Experiments on conscious, freely breathing dogs have shown that central and peripheral chemoreceptors are interdependent in regulating pH and PCO_2, and that chemoreceptors of the carotid bodies contribute more than 50 percent of the total drive for physiological breathing.

As well as being responsive to elevations in carbon dioxide in the blood and to metabolic acidosis, respiratory chemoreceptors are sensitive to hypoglycemia (low blood sugar), hyperthermia (elevated body temperature), hyperosmolarity (excess concentrations of osmotically active chemicals), and hyperkalemia (elevated potassium in the blood). These metabolic stimuli activate the carotid bodies, causing release of excitatory neuro-transmitters that increase the frequency and intensity of the excitatory signals reaching respiratory and cardiovascular control centers in the brainstem. Moreover, the carotid bodies are the initial and probably the more influential responders to hypoxia. The usual reflex responses to these and related metabolic signals are hyperventilation, reduced heart rate, and peripheral vasoconstriction. All of these changes result from the increased discharge of motor neurons in the phrenic, intercostal, sympa-thetic (except for heart rate), and parasympathetic nerves. These chemi-cally sensitive reflexes maintain respiratory homeostasis by matching ventilation to the metabolic production of carbon dioxide and organic acids (for example, lactic acid) that are produced throughout the body.

Several changes in the way elderly subjects breathe at rest and during activity compensate for alterations in compliance and gas exchange as they age. For example, elderly subjects maintain alveolar ventilation at the same approximate level as young adults by breathing more rapidly at lower tidal volumes. During exercise, the respiratory response to elevated levels of carbon dioxide is greater in the elderly than in young adults, even though the same levels of physiological PCO_2 are maintained in both age groups. Also during exposure to elevations in carbon dioxide, the thresh-old for increased inspiration is reduced as we age. This means that it takes a smaller increase in PCO_2 in the elderly to stimulate increased ventilation. Alas, older subjects are less able to detect increases in the resistance against which they breathe than are younger subjects. Therefore, they do not compensate for increased resistance as well as younger people do.

The increased frequency of breathing that maintains alveolar ventila-tion and PCO_2 in the elderly at the same approximate levels as in young adults is most likely an adaptation that developed to counteract the reduc-tion in age-related tidal volume. Changes in the reactivity and function of central chemoreceptors and peripheral mechanoreceptors have been pro-posed as the cause, but that theory has not been substantiated. Readjust-ments in the cerebral cortex that help maintain respiratory frequency and minute ventilation in proportion to changes in PCO_2 might also be involved. This is thought to be the case because the input and output connections in the cerebral cortex that influence respiration have been identified by functional magnetic resonance images (MRIs) in young adults. In addition, studies in the elderly that examined cortical control of breathing showed that when spontaneous respiration was replaced by a voluntarily paced breathing, minute ventilation was maintained to keep pace with changes in carbon dioxide, dead space ventilation, and metabolic rate.

If the cerebral cortex is a controller that helps adjust the frequency of breathing, how are the nerve circuits arranged, and do they change with age? Studies on humans provide few answers to these and related questions, but experiments on cats have found nerve tracts that project from the cerebral cortex and spinal cord directly into the phrenic and intercostal motor neurons. Since these direct projections bypass brainstem centers that generate respiratory rhythms and patterns, it seems likely that the higher central nervous system pathways influence tidal volume but not breathing frequency. Moreover, activation of neurons in deep cerebellar nuclei of the cat and in the hypothalamus of the rat (near the cerebral ventricles) increases the firing frequency and intensity of the phrenic nerve. Still other studies in animals show that there are several parallel neuronal pathways that influence rhythmic motor output and have connections with the cerebral cortex.

During exercise, the amount of carbon dioxide that we breathe out at the end of expiration (end tidal CO_2) is lower in the elderly than in young adults. This is true even when the two age groups are exercising at the same level of intensity. The amount of carbon dioxide in expired air is a common way of identifying hyper- or hypoventilation. Increased ventilation during exercise in the elderly is accompanied by little or no change in end tidal CO_2 and compensates for a greater volume of dead space. However, the ventilatory response to exercise estimated from the ratio of the volume of air moved to the amount of CO_2 expelled is greater in older people. In young adults, alterations in the function of peripheral chemoreceptors is not a factor in the ventilatory response to exercise. However, reactivity to changes of carbon dioxide in cerebral blood (central chemoreceptors) in young adults increases during exercise. So far no similar reports are available for elderly subjects during exercise.

The CO_2 threshold for increased inspiratory effort is lower in the elderly, and there are no known neuronal mechanisms that explain why.

Some investigators think that it might be a compensatory response to off-set an increase in PCO_2 in the central nervous system. The compensation could be triggered by reduced cerebral blood flow, resulting in higher tissue levels of CO_2 near central chemoreceptors. Also, there is general agreement that decreased perception of increased resistance during inspiration occurs in the elderly, and that coughs are less powerful and productive. One reason for the latter is that the sensation to cough is suppressed. The reduced sensitivity to irritants among the aging seems to involve several factors, including reduced tone of bronchiolar smooth muscle, elevated thresholds to stimulation in vagal sensory nerve fibers, and impaired perception in the cerebral cortex. Since strength of the respiratory muscles normally decreases with age, the motor component of the cough reflex that is essential for clearing the airways might also be less effective. Thus, the weakened cough reflex could be a factor in the higher incidence of aspiration pneumonia in older people.

Respiratory Sensitivity to Hypercapnia and Hypoxia with Age

Standard methods for evaluating sensitivity to elevated carbon dioxide (hypercapnia) and to reduced oxygen (hypoxia) in humans include measuring breathing patterns using spirometers and/or plethysmographs and measuring pressure in the mouth while manipulating alveolar carbon dioxide and/or oxygen. Respiratory responses to elevated carbon dioxide have been studied extensively in nonhuman animals and other experimental preparations. The usual response to increased carbon dioxide is an increase in the amount of air taken in, which is caused primarily by increasing tidal volume. This means that we breathe deeper during hypercapnia. In adult humans whose sinus nerves have been severed (accidentally or surgically), central responsiveness to elevations in carbon dioxide or to reductions in pH are impaired. Following surgery, the ventilatory response to hypercapnia is temporarily reduced, reaching a steady state after three to six months and then slowly returning to presurgical levels within two years.

The sensitivity to hypoxia-induced hyperventilation in younger adults depends on the relative degree of hypoxia and the methods used to induce it. Exposure of young adults to transient, moderate hypoxia increases the duration of inspiration and tidal volume, whereas the duration of expiration does not change significantly. In male young adults exposed over several days to moderate periodic hypoxia with normal levels of carbon dioxide, tidal volume increases to a plateau within one to four days without a significant change in respiratory frequency. When a single episode of moderate hypoxia (with normal carbon dioxide) is maintained for twenty to thirty minutes, minute ventilation rises to a peak for several minutes, then declines over the next twenty minutes to about 50 percent of the peak increase. Repeated episodes of moderate hypoxia lasting three to five minutes each and interrupted by bouts of normoxia evoke a progressive increase in respiratory motor output during normoxic periods. This is referred to as "facilitation," and it might persist for an hour after episodes of hypoxia. During facilitation, the frequency of breathing but not the tidal volume is increased. Similar experiments have not been performed in older adults, so we do not know how age might affect facilitation.

Severe hypoxia (for example, PO_2 in venous blood of $\leqslant 8$–10 mmHg; physiological levels are $\geqslant 40$ mmHg) maintained over several minutes causes a biphasic respiratory response in humans as well as in other mammals. Initial augmentation of ventilation (driven by the carotid bodies) is followed by cessation of breathing (apnea) and gasping. The latter are mediated by the central nervous system and respiratory control centers in the brainstem. Severing of nerves leading from the peripheral chemoreceptors selectively eliminates the initial augmentation. However, the mechanisms responsible for apnea and gasping during severe acute hypoxia are complex.

Hypoxia-induced depression of respiratory and other nerves is associated with decreasing stores of intracellular energy and other responses that are designed to conserve energy and postpone cell death. In respiratory regions of the brainstem of the cat, concentrations of glutamate and other neurotransmitters increase during the initial augmentation of respiration, then decrease during apnea. Conversely, chemicals such as serotonin and adenosine gradually increase with the onset of depression. Both of these agents are vasoactive and might increase to compensate for the lack of oxygen in the blood. That is, by increasing blood flow (vasodilation), even during hypoxia, more oxygen will be delivered to the tissues than if blood flow remained stable.

Most investigators report significant reductions in respiratory sensitivity to elevated carbon dioxide and reduced oxygen in elderly subjects. When researchers estimated airway resistance to hyperventilation (reduced carbon dioxide in expired air), they found no significant difference between elderly and young subjects. However, under concomitant hypoxic conditions, airway resistance during hyperventilation increased in young but not in older adults. Elderly subjects had lower oral pressure responses to hypoxia and hypercapnia, while there was a progressive, age-related decrease in threshold sensitivity when alveolar PCO_2 was increased. Compared to younger subjects, in the elderly responses of oral pressure to hypoxia at physiological levels of carbon dioxide were reduced by about 50 percent, and to elevated carbon dioxide in the presence of excess oxygen by about 60 percent. Ventilatory responses to both excess carbon dioxide and low oxygen were lower in aged subjects, due primarily to reduced neuromuscular effort during inspiration. It seems likely that the attenuation of ventilatory drive during elevated carbon dioxide and reduced oxygen in elderly humans involves both diminished chemosensory function and structural changes in the lungs and chest wall that reduce motor performance.

Other Aging-Related Changes in Breathing

During sleep that is characterized by nonrapid eye movements (non-REM sleep), the amplitudes and frequency of breathing are regular in all healthy adults regardless of age. During non-REM sleep, minute ventilation decreases by about 15 percent, and mean inspiratory flow rate and tidal volume decrease modestly when compared with waking hours. Three-dimensional displacement of the rib cage decreases, abdominal contractility increases slightly, and contractility of the diaphragm remains unchanged.

During sleep that is characterized by rapid eye movements (REM sleep), airflow and tidal volume are highly variable. Changes in the central regulation of respiration during REM sleep cause irregularities in tidal volume and respiratory frequency, as well as periodic apnea. The above sleep-related changes in breathing can result in hypoventilation, hypercapnia, and hypoxia. Resistance in the upper airways increases during sleep because of reductions in tone in the pharyngeal dilator muscles partial collapse of the airways.

In the elderly as well as in younger adults, respiratory responsiveness to elevated carbon dioxide is attenuated during sleep. This means that in either age group there is an incremental elevation in the amount of carbon dioxide in expired air during the transition from wakefulness to non-REM and then to REM sleep. The change can be as much as 5 mmHg PCO_2 during REM sleep. Also in the elderly, sensitivity of central chemoreceptors to changes in pH and carbon dioxide decreases, as does the motor activity of chest, neck, and upper airway muscles. Fortunately for the elderly and those around them, sleep apnea has no immediately negative consequences with respect to alertness, mobility, mood, and temperament. Unfortunately, hypoxia-induced sleep apnea can promote the development of new blood vessels (angiogenesis). In healthy tissues this can be a good thing, resulting in improved delivery of oxygen in times of need, but it can also lead to growth of tumors and to higher incidence of mortality from cancer.

Compared to younger adults, elderly subjects spend less time in REM sleep, but more time in light and slow-wave sleep. In addition, sleep-related circadian rhythms are weaker, more desynchronized, and less prominent in the aging. Thus, the quality of sleep decreases as we age. Factors proposed to account for these aging-related changes include the reduced secretion of melatonin (a factor in the regulation of diurnal rhythms) and neural degeneration. Obstructive sleep apnea, central sleep apnea, and periodic breathing characterized by recurring episodes of increasing followed by decreasing tidal volumes and minute ventilation (Cheyne-Stokes respiration) also occur more frequently in the elderly than in young adults.

Elderly subjects are more sensitive to respiratory depression by opioids and sedative hypnotics. This results from aging-related changes in responses to drugs. Most drugs are distributed and metabolized more slowly in the elderly. Circulating concentrations of drugs increase as we age because their volumes of distribution decrease, due to reductions in lean muscle mass, total body water, and excretion by the kidneys. Decreased glomerular filtration in the kidneys and reduced blood flow to the liver compromise the body's capacity to excrete pain-relieving opioids, sedative hypnotics, and their metabolites. This, in turn, prolongs both the toxic and the therapeutic effects of the drugs. It can also cause episodic waxing and waning of effective breathing, insufficient ventilation, and poor gas exchange. Neither cause-effect relationships nor the neural mechanisms are fully understood, but ineffective chemical feedback control has been suggested as a contributing factor.

The effects of aging on ventilation and breathing are progressive and gradual. The major changes emanate from the degeneration of respiratory structures particularly, as they affect the lungs, chest wall, glottis, and upper airways (trachea and major bronchi). Breathing patterns in the elderly adjust to structural deterioration through adaptations in the respiratory control centers of the medulla and brainstem. This helps maintain effective pulmonary gas exchange even if an inequality in the ventilation-to-perfusion ratio progresses. Whereas aging-related structure-function relationships that directly involve the airways and respiratory pump (that is, the thorax) are well known and easily explained, changes in the brainstem and higher neuronal networks largely remain a mystery. More work is needed.

INDEX

Page numbers in *italics* refer to tables.

ABOUT THE AUTHOR

GARY F. MERRILL is a professor in the Department of Cell Biology and Neuroscience, Division of Life Sciences, at Rutgers University. He earned his BS, MS, and PhD degrees in classic mammalian physiology. He teaches juniors and seniors who are interested in medical or graduate school and manages a research laboratory that focuses on cardiovascular physiology. Among his hobbies are family outings, hiking and camping, and taking care of cars.